AF668367

Review of AIIMS May 2017

Review of AIIMS May 2017

With Explanatory Answers
(Including Image-Based Questions)

Mukesh Bhatia
Senior Consultant, Physician
Fortis Hospital, Delhi, India
Director, DBMCI
New Delhi, India

Edited By
DBMCI PREMIER FACULTY

JAYPEE The Health Sciences Publisher
New Delhi | London | Panama |

JAYPEE **Jaypee Brothers Medical Publishers (P) Ltd**

Headquarters

Jaypee Brothers Medical Publishers (P) Ltd.
4838/24, Ansari Road, Daryaganj
New Delhi 110 002, India
Phone: +91-11-43574357
Fax: +91-11-43574314
Email: jaypee@jaypeebrothers.com

Overseas Offices

J.P. Medical Ltd.
83, Victoria Street, London
SW1H 0HW (UK)
Phone: +44-20 3170 8910
Fax: +44-(0)20 3008 6180
Email: info@jpmedpub.com

Jaypee-Highlights Medical Publishers Inc.
City of Knowledge, Bld. 235, 2nd Floor, Clayton
Panama City, Panama
Phone: +1 507-301-0496
Fax: +1 507-301-0499
Email: cservice@jphmedical.com

Jaypee Brothers Medical Publishers (P) Ltd.
17/1-B, Babar Road, Block-B, Shaymali
Mohammadpur, Dhaka-1207, Bangladesh
Mobile: +08801912003485
Email: jaypeedhaka@gmail.com

Jaypee Brothers Medical Publishers (P) Ltd.
Bhotahity, Kathmandu, Nepal
Phone: +977-9741283608
Email: kathmandu@jaypeebrothers.com

Website: www.jaypeebrothers.com
Website: www.jaypeedigital.com

© 2017, Jaypee Brothers Medical Publishers

The views and opinions expressed in this book are solely those of the original contributor(s)/author(s) and do not necessarily represent those of editor(s) of the book.

All rights reserved. No part of this publication may be reproduced, stored or transmitted in any form or by any means, electronic, mechanical, photocopying, recording or otherwise, without the prior permission in writing of the publishers.

All brand names and product names used in this book are trade names, service marks, trademarks or registered trademarks of their respective owners. The publisher is not associated with any product or vendor mentioned in this book.

Medical knowledge and practice change constantly. This book is designed to provide accurate, authoritative information about the subject matter in question. However, readers are advised to check the most current information available on procedures included and check information from the manufacturer of each product to be administered, to verify the recommended dose, formula, method and duration of administration, adverse effects and contraindications. It is the responsibility of the practitioner to take all appropriate safety precautions. Neither the publisher nor the author(s)/editor(s) assume any liability for any injury and/or damage to persons or property arising from or related to use of material in this book.

This book is sold on the understanding that the publisher is not engaged in providing professional medical services. If such advice or services are required, the services of a competent medical professional should be sought.

Every effort has been made where necessary to contact holders of copyright to obtain permission to reproduce copyright material. If any have been inadvertently overlooked, the publisher will be pleased to make the necessary arrangements at the first opportunity.

Inquiries for bulk sales may be solicited at: jaypee@jaypeebrothers.com

Review of AIIMS May 2017

First Edition: **2017**

ISBN: 978-93-5270-141-4

Printed at Rajkamal Electric Press, Plot No. 2, Phase-IV, Kundli, Haryana.

Review Board

S. No.	Subject	Faculty
1.	ANATOMY	Dr Ashwani Kumar, Dr Manisha Hansda
2.	PHYSIOLOGY	Dr Ashish, Dr Soumen
3.	BIOCHEMISTRY	Dr Nilesh Chandra, Dr Smiley
4.	PATHOLOGY	Dr Praveen Kumar, Dr Vandana Puri, Dr Sushant Soni, Dr Sanjay Saxena
5.	PHARMACOLOGY	Dr Saurabh Bhatia, Dr Ankit Kumar, Dr Arpit Aggarwal
6.	MICROBIOLOGY	Dr Shivika Juneja, Dr Sonu Panwar
7.	FORENSIC MEDICINE	Dr Gurudutta, Dr Atul Kumar, Dr Sumit Tellwar
8.	ORTHOPAEDICS	Dr Sushil Vijay, Dr Mukul Anand
9.	OPHTHALMOLOGY	Dr Ray, Dr Utsav, Dr Neha, Dr Pulkit Gupta
10.	ENT	Dr Sanjay Agarwal, Dr Darwin Kaushal
11.	PSM	Dr Madhu, Dr Anshul Shukla
12.	MEDICINE	Dr Mukesh Bhatia, Dr Thameem Saif, Dr Rajat Bajaj, Dr Akshay Bafna
13.	SURGERY	Dr Jai, Dr Sujoy Neogi, Dr Rakesh Mittal
14.	PAEDIATRICS	Dr Sanjay Khatri, Dr Pankaj Tikku, Dr Deepak Gupta
15.	OBS & GYNE	Dr Prassan Vij, Dr Monika Nagpal
16.	DERMATOLOGY	Dr Manish Soni
17.	ANAESTHESIA	Dr Swati, Dr Amit Kohli, Dr Ajay Yadav
18.	RADIOLOGY	Dr Rajat Jain
19.	PSYCHIATRY	Dr Sandeep Govil, Dr Praveen Tripathi

Preface

This book is primarily meant for those students who are preparing for AIIMS PG Entrance Exams. Our effort to come up with this current book is due to huge demand by AIIMS aspirants who are in search of quality book with genuine recall of questions with correct options and most authentic answers with relevant references. Every solved question will have a valid reference citing a standard textbook or article in order to increase the credibility of the answers. The focussed explanations should help you solve questions from same topics in the future easily. Our book would serve as a true companion for all those hard working PG Aspirants with most authentic answers from highly reputed faculties. For making the book authentic we needed crisp explanations and authentic referencing, explaining the picture based questions, each requiring expertise. The only solution was to seek help. Every chapter in this book was solved by the masters in their own subjects.

We have incorporated a systematic approach in solving each and every question which can be appreciated while reading this book. We have tried to put our best effort to give correct explanations in the right contexts covering maximum topics.

The schematic diagrams, tables, illustrations, bulleted key points and references are highlights of this book and will make reading and understanding of the material easier and effective.

All the information have been presented in a point-wise manner making it easy to remember and revise. All these questions have been solved by subject faculty of DBMCI. This is the most important point about the book unlike other books which are written by a single author, writing a book on 19 subjects. Hence, similar books by other authors have a lot of mistakes and they are not updated also.

Hope we are able to provide you a quality book which can go a long way in helping you preparing for upcoming AIIMS and other PGMEE exams. We hope the students will find this book very useful. Your comments, feedback and suggestions are welcome on our facebook group **"DBMCI 2017 Premiere Group" or in E-mail id: studentsupport@dbmi.edu.in**

Our Job does not end here with providing you with the book. We also want to help you throughout your journey. So, we have a created a **Facebook Premiere Group** i.e. **"DBMCI 2017 Premiere Group" on Facebook** which is purely intended to help you all. This group aims to cater to the students directly, in discussing the updates in various subjects related to PG Entrance Exams and solving queries/ doubts pertaining to all the subjects of PG Entrance Exams within 2 hours. You can join it using following link.

https://www.facebook.com/groups/1769262746733609/

Wishing you all the best for a bright future!!!!

Best Wishes
Mukesh Bhatia
Director, DBMCI
Website: www.dbmci.com
E-mail: studentsupport@dbmi.edu.in

Acknowledgments

First of all I thank **Lord Krishna** for teaching me the concept of **Gyan Yoga** (importance of always Learning) and **Karam Yoga** (to do one's duty with utmost sincerity - Work is Worship!!!).

I am thankful to **Lord Ganpati** whose eternal blessings, divine presence and masterly guidance helps all of us to fulfil our Goals.

I am thankful to **My Mother and (Late) Father** for their constant undemanding love, dedication, sacrifice, inspiring guidance, affectionate encouragement and never-ending enthusiasm; without which this book would not have seen the light of the day.

I would like to thank all the faculty of DBMCI for their commitment and hard work throughout the process. I would also like to thank our publishing and Academics team:

1. **Dr Manish Hansda (MD, Anatomy)**
2. **Mr Kuldeep Bisht (Academic Manager)**

For their rentless efforts in releasing this book in a short notice, who worked at odd hours to make the book a visual treat.

We are looking forward to hearing your feedback and are fully committed in bringing out better Editions in the future.

Write to us:

Any Observation, suggestions, feedbacks are welcome at: studentsupport@dbmi.edu.in

Follow us on Facebook:

https://www.facebook.com/dbmci/?ref=bookmarks

Mukesh Bhatia
Director, DBMCI
30th May 2017, New Delhi

DR BHATIA
MEDICAL COACHING INSTITUTE
Estd. 1996 No.1 PG Medical Coaching Institute Of India

HALL OF FAME

Another perfect score in AIIMS May 2017

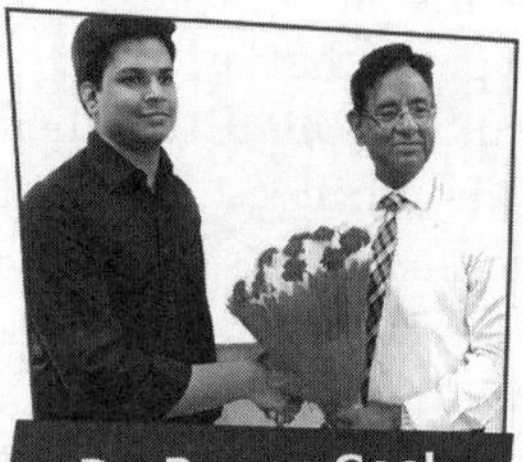
Dr. Pawan Goel
Rank - 1

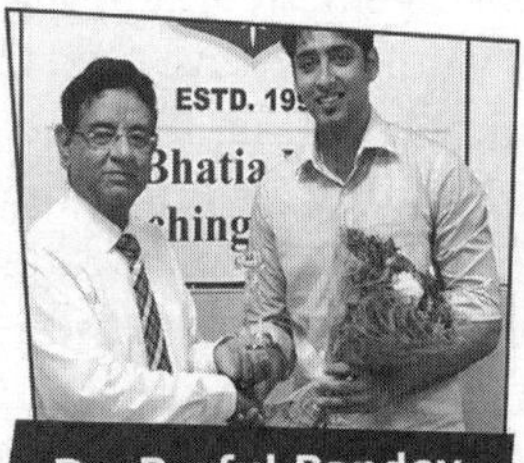
Dr. Praful Pandey
Rank - 2

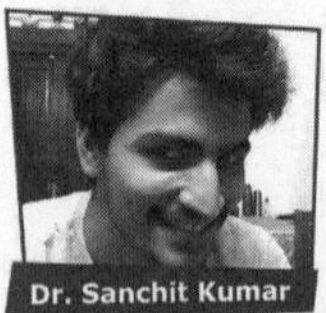
Dr. Sanchit Kumar
Rank - 3

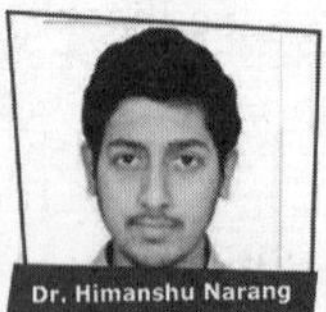
Dr. Himanshu Narang
Rank - 4

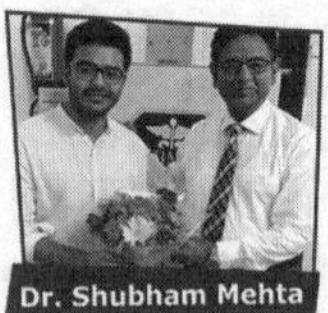
Dr. Shubham Mehta
Rank - 5

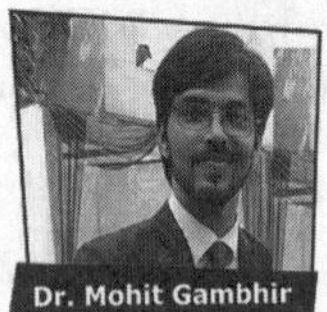
Dr. Mohit Gambhir
Rank - 6

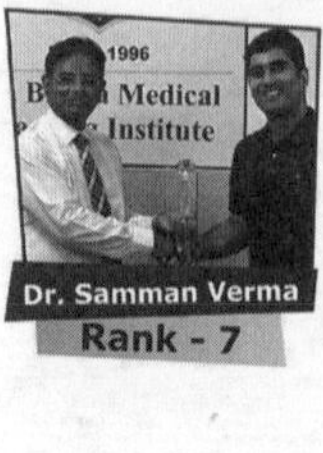
Dr. Samman Verma
Rank - 7

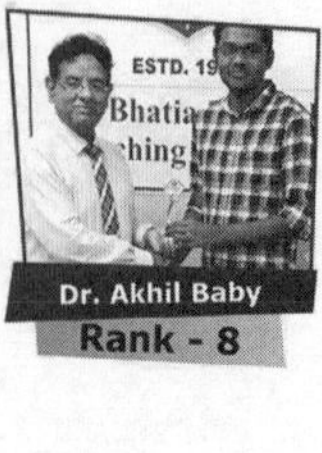
Dr. Akhil Baby
Rank - 8

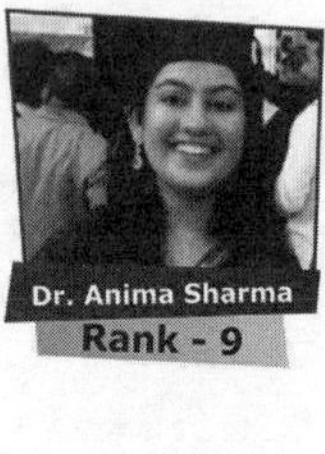
Dr. Anima Sharma
Rank - 9

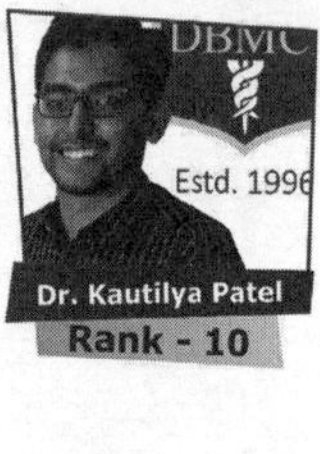
Dr. Kautilya Patel
Rank - 10

DR BHATIA
MEDICAL COACHING INSTITUTE
Estd. 1996 No.1 PG Medical Coaching Institute Of India

HALL OF FAME

PGI May 2017

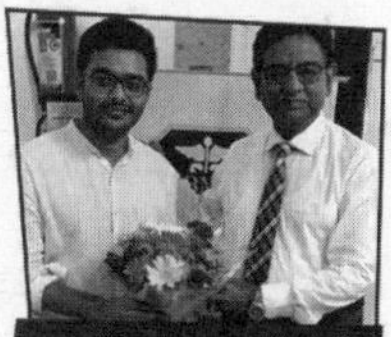
Dr. Shubham Mehta
Rank - 1

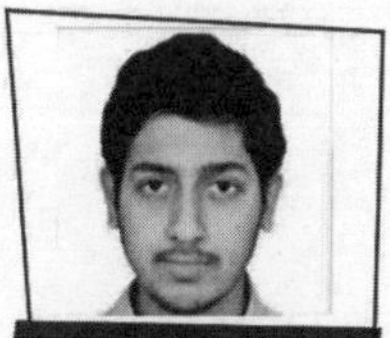
Dr. Himanshu Narang
Rank - 2

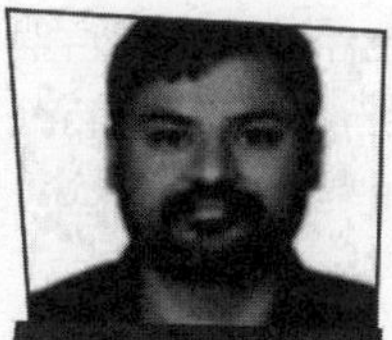
Dr. Kesha Meghashyma
Rank - 3

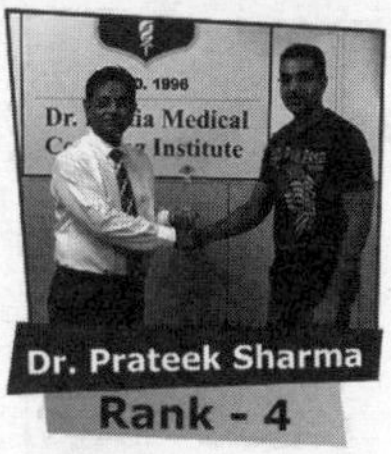
Dr. Prateek Sharma
Rank - 4

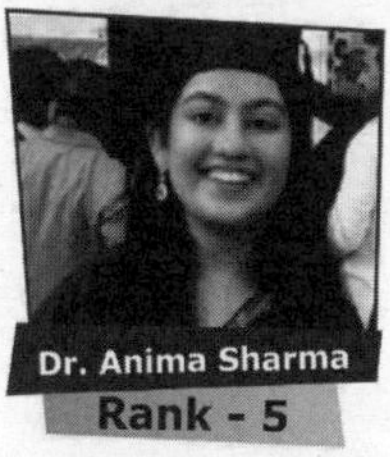
Dr. Anima Sharma
Rank - 5

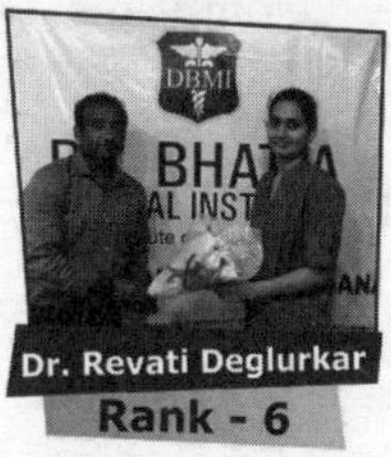
Dr. Revati Deglurkar
Rank - 6

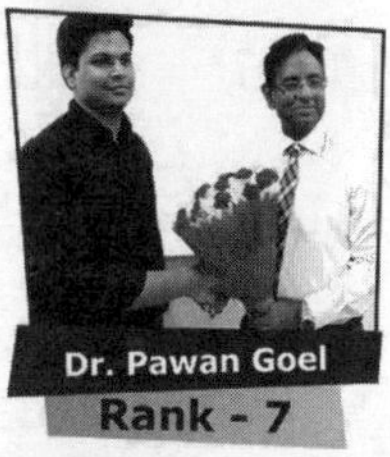
Dr. Pawan Goel
Rank - 7

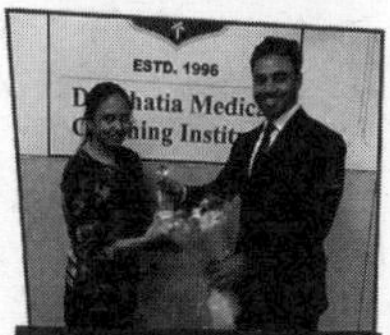
Dr. Rupali Jain
Rank - 8

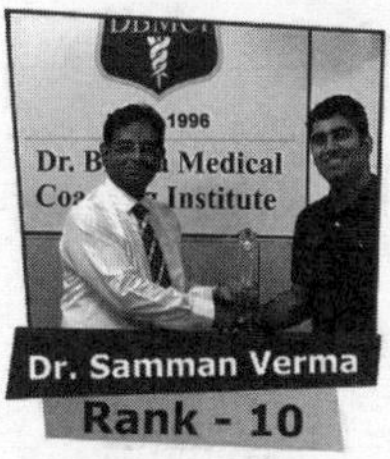
Dr. Samman Verma
Rank - 10

Your Success is Our Motto

Contents

Color Plates

PLATE 1

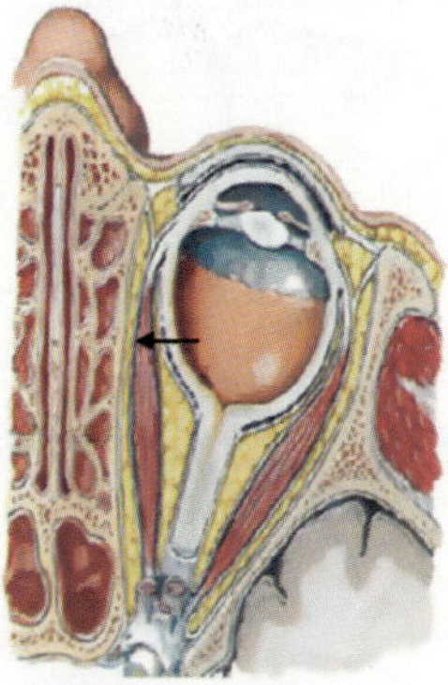

Chapter 1. Figure 1: Q 6

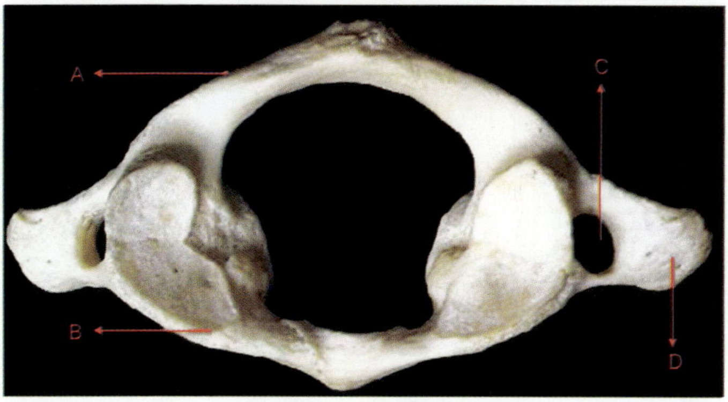

Chapter 1. Figure 2: Q 7

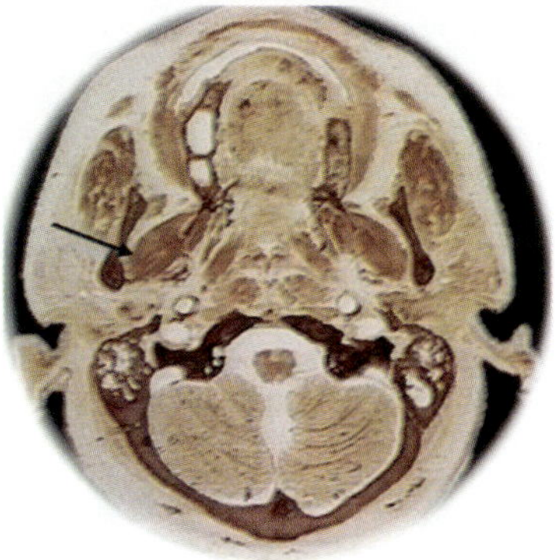

Chapter 1. Figure 3: Q 8

PLATE 2

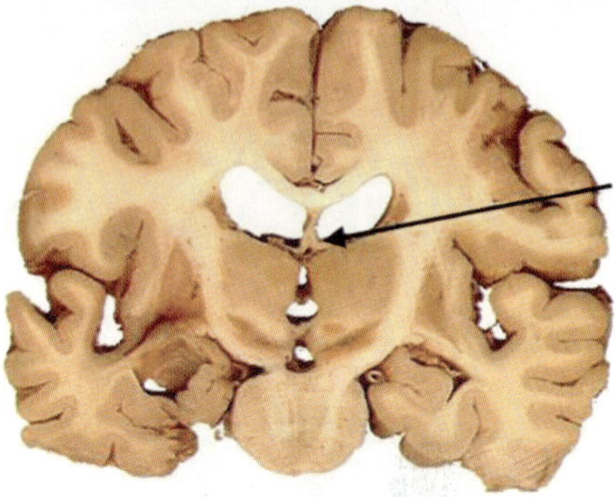

Chapter 1. Figure 4: Q 9

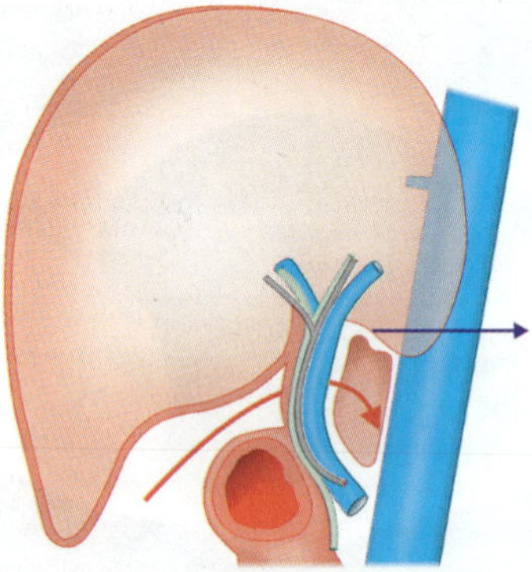

Chapter 1. Figure 5: Q 10

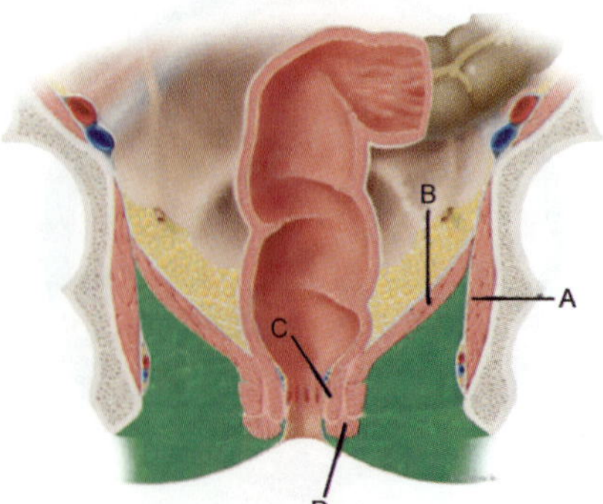

Chapter 1. Figure 6: Q 11

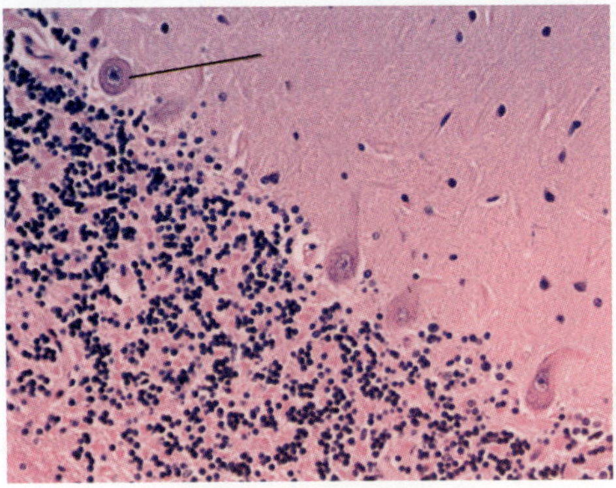

Chapter 1. Figure 7: Q 12

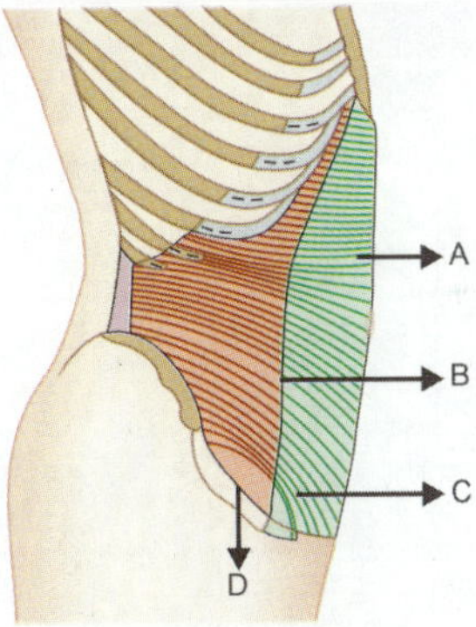

Chapter 1. Figure 8: Q 13

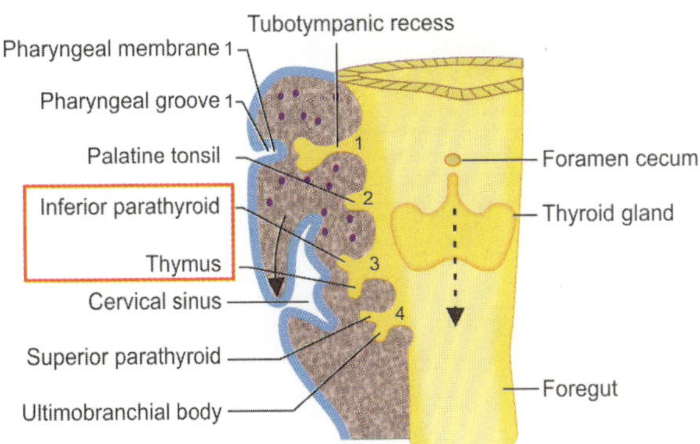

Chapter 1. Figure 9: Ans. 1

PLATE 4

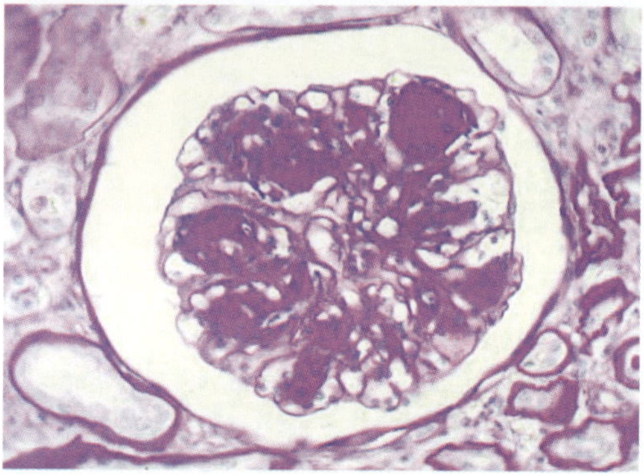

Chapter 4. Figure 10: Q 1

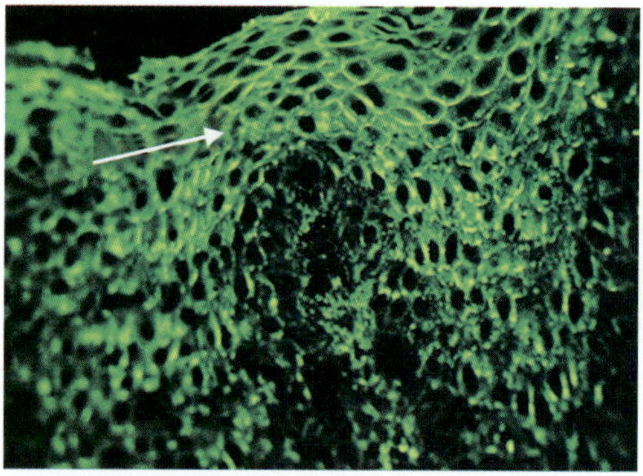

Chapter 4. Figure 11: Q 2

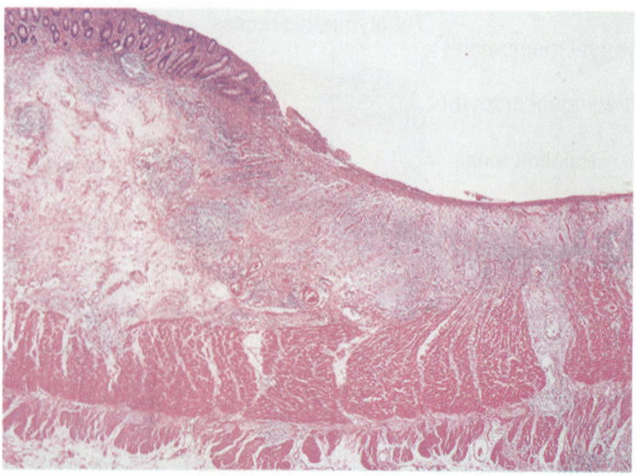

Chapter 4. Figure 12: Q 5

PLATE 5

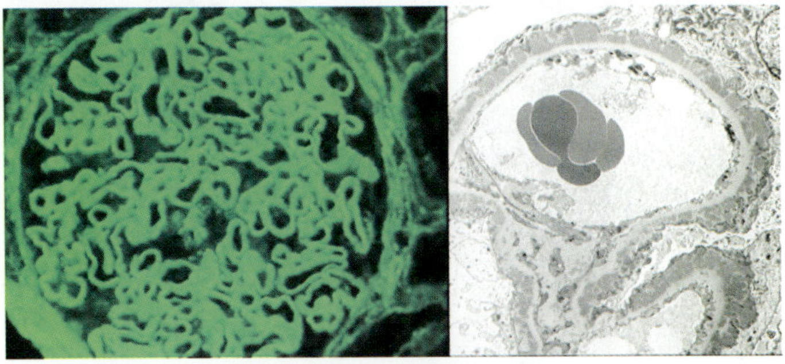

Chapter 4. Figure 13: Q 15

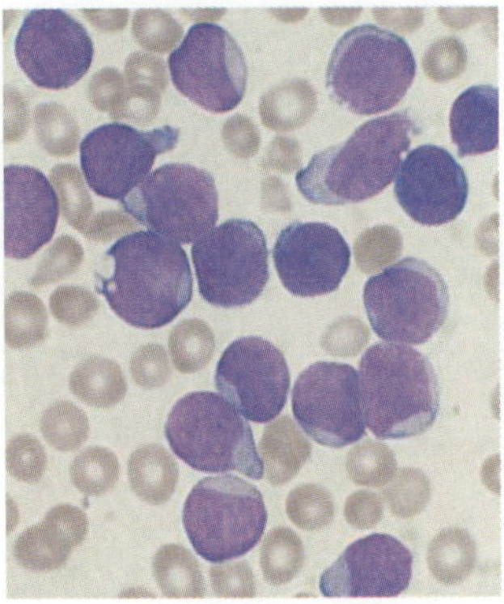

Chapter 4. Figure 14: Q 16

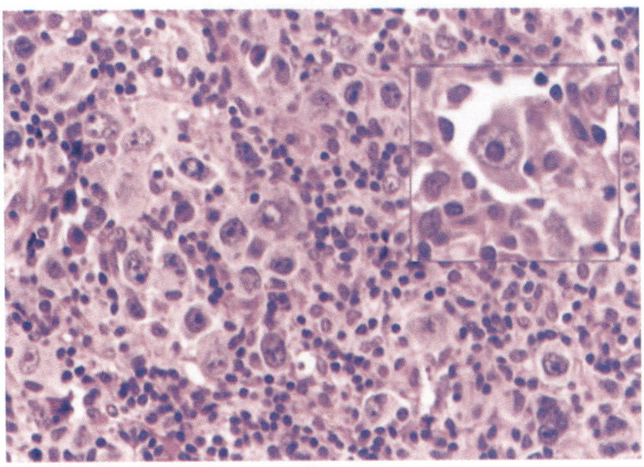

Chapter 4. Figure 15: Q 17

PLATE 6

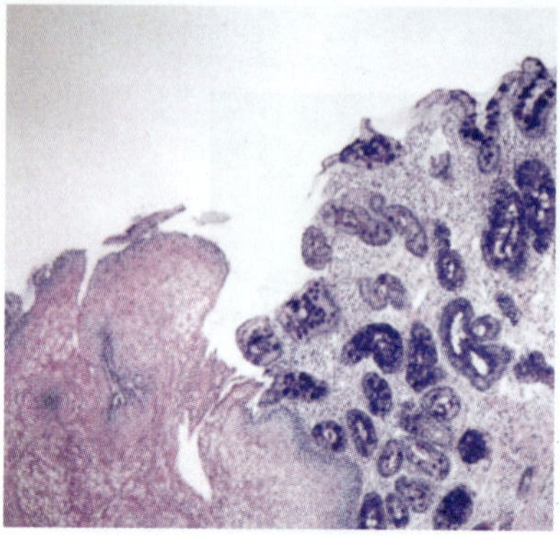

Chapter 4. Figure 16: Q 18

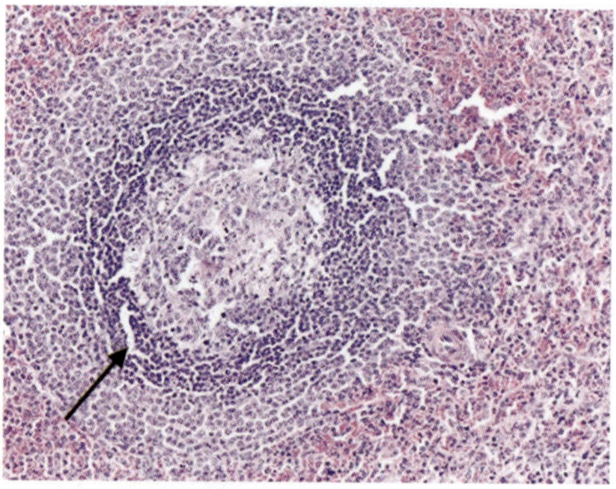

Chapter 4. Figure 17: Q 21

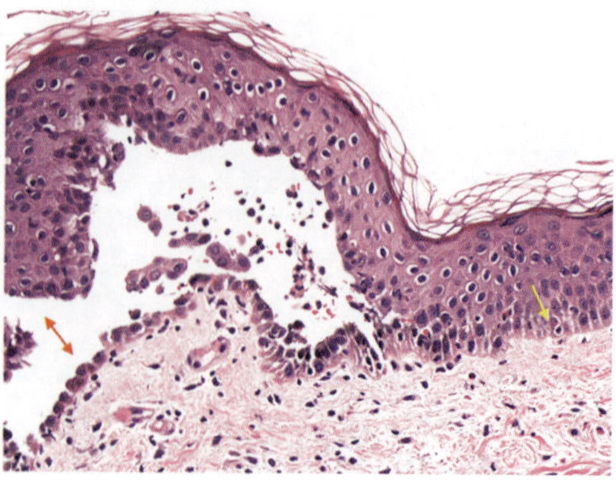

Chapter 4. Figure 18: Q 26

PLATE 7

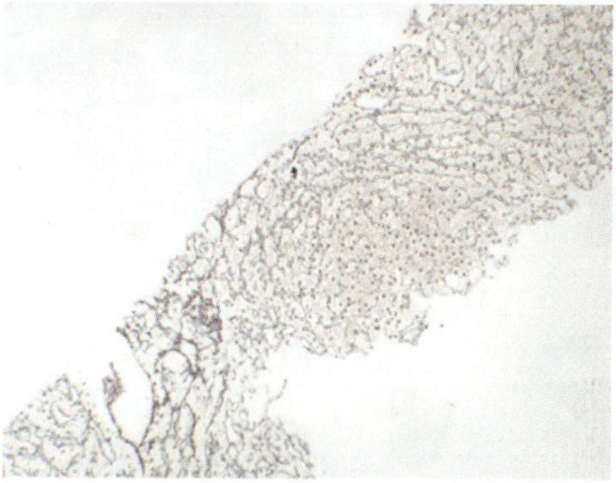

Chapter 4. Figure 19: Q 27

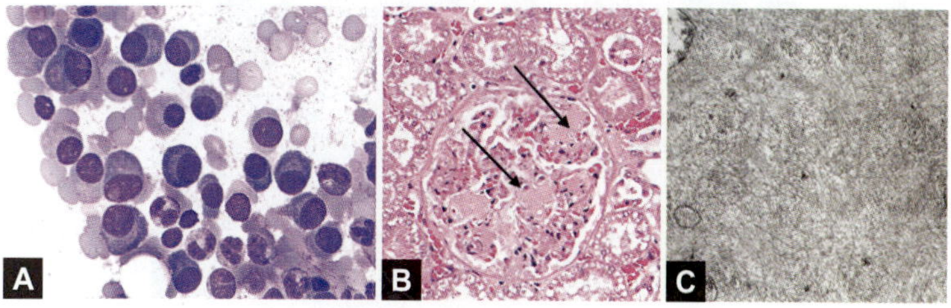

Chapter 4. Figure 20: Q 28

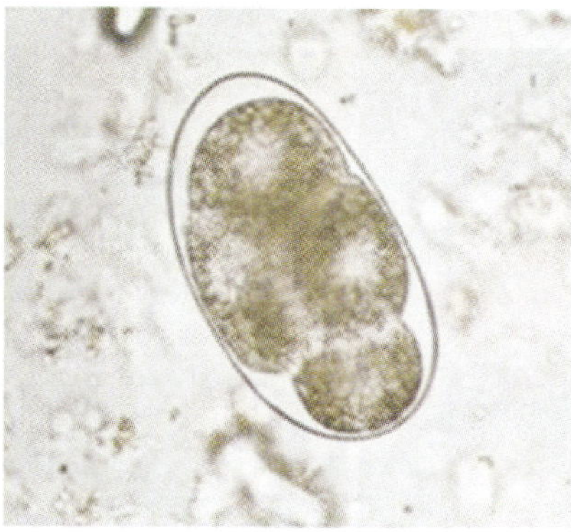

Chapter 6. Figure 21: Q 3

PLATE 8

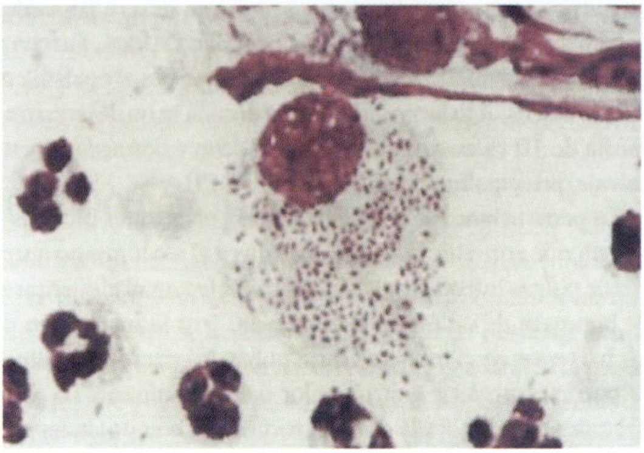

Chapter 6. Figure 22: Q 4

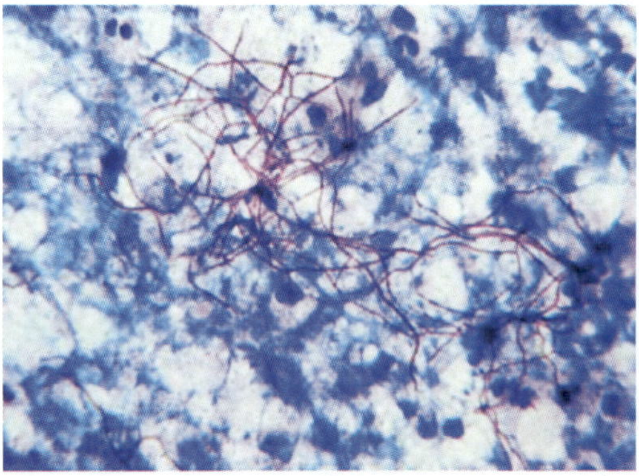

Chapter 6. Figure 23: Q 6

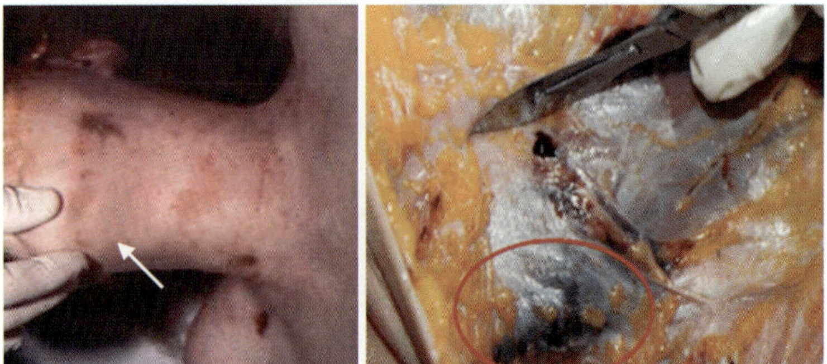

Chapter 7. Figure 24: Q 7

PLATE 9

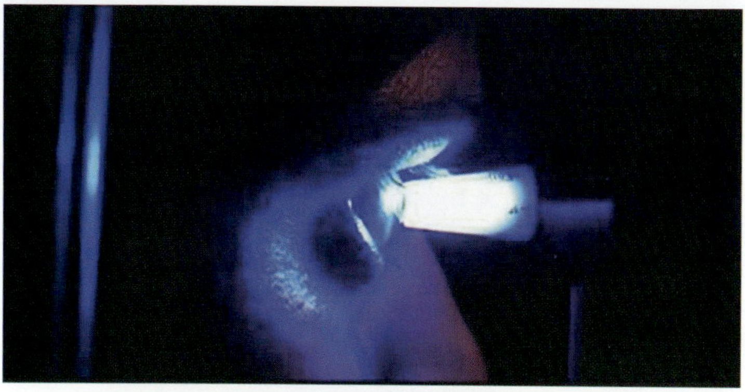

Chapter 9. Figure 25: Q 1

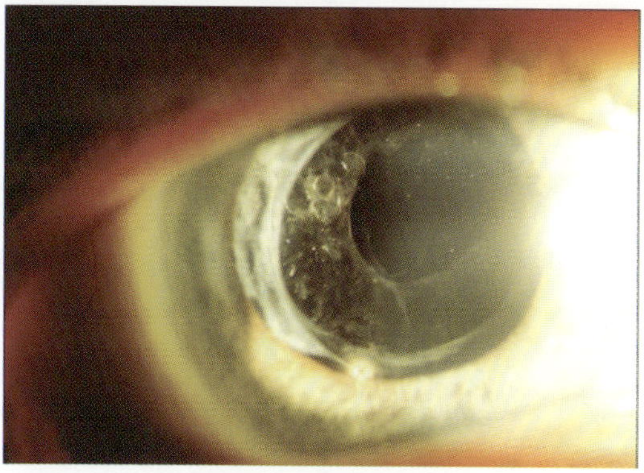

Chapter 9. Figure 26: Q 2

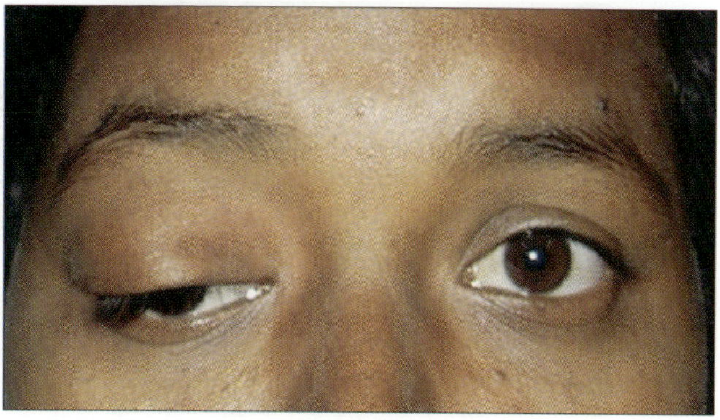

Chapter 9. Figure 27: Q 4

PLATE 10

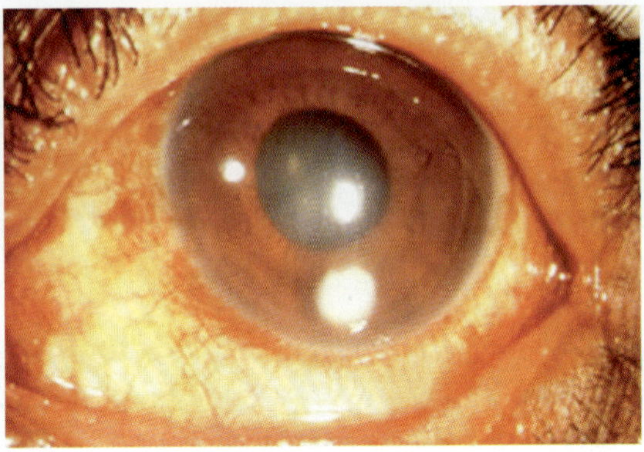

Chapter 9. Figure 28: Q 6

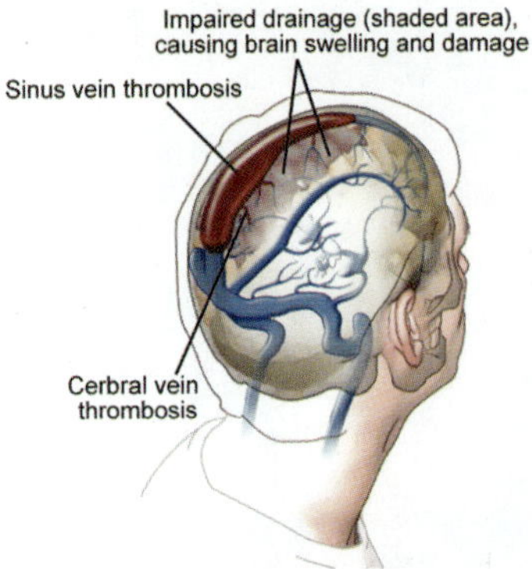

Chapter 12. Figure 29: Q 18

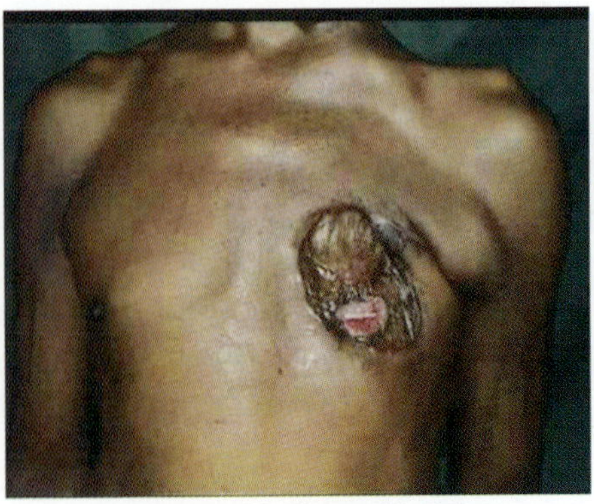

Chapter 13. Figure 30: Q 8

PLATE 11

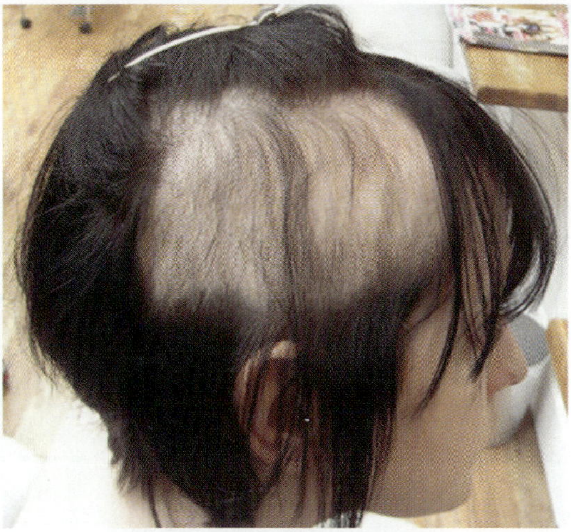

Chapter 16. Figure 31: Q 1

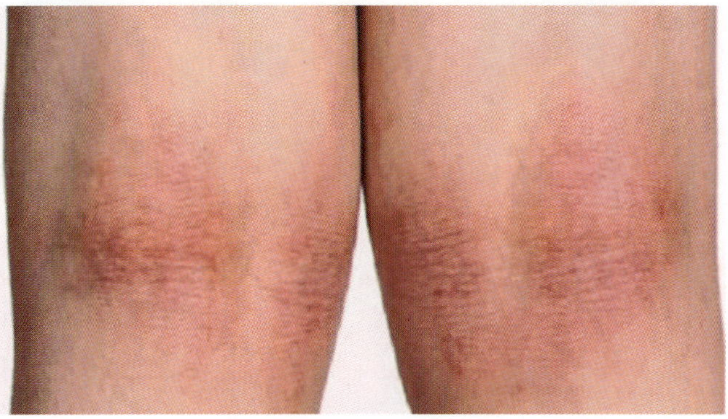

Chapter 16. Figure 32: Q 2

PLATE 12

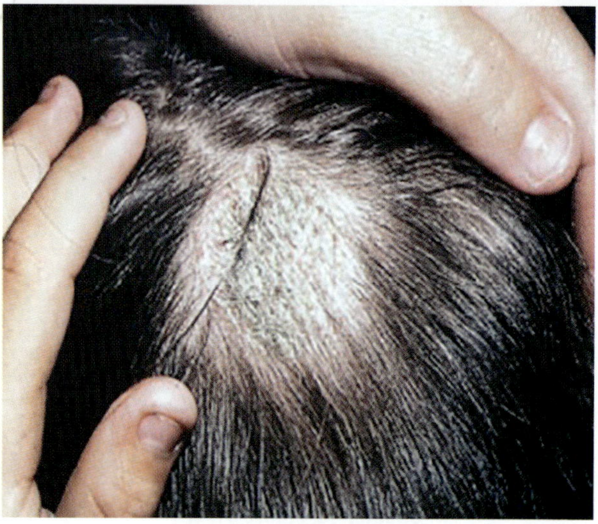

Chapter 16. Figure 33: Q 3

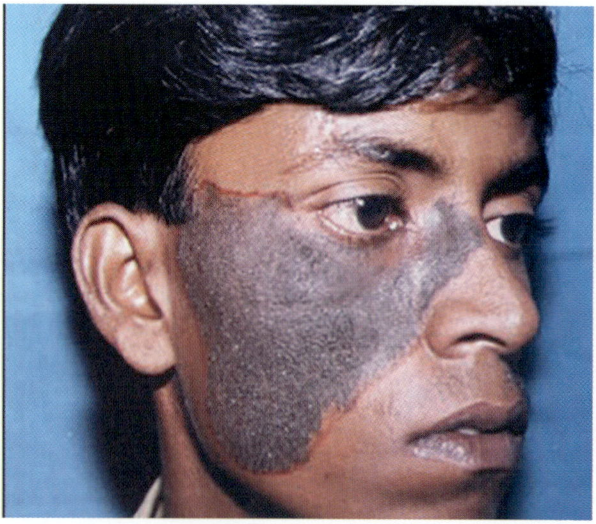

Chapter 16. Figure 34: Q 4

ANATOMY

QUESTIONS

1. A young patient with absent thymus and presented with hypoparathyroidism and tetany. Which of the following marked areas in the picture is defective in this condition?

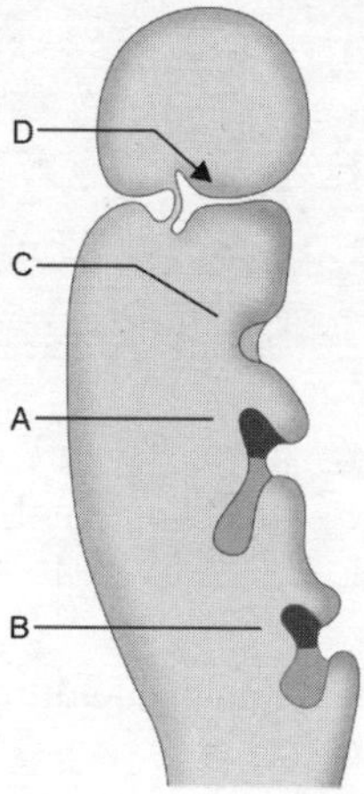

a. A	b. B
c. C	d. D

2. Which of the following structures in the scapula is palpable in the infraclavicular fossa?

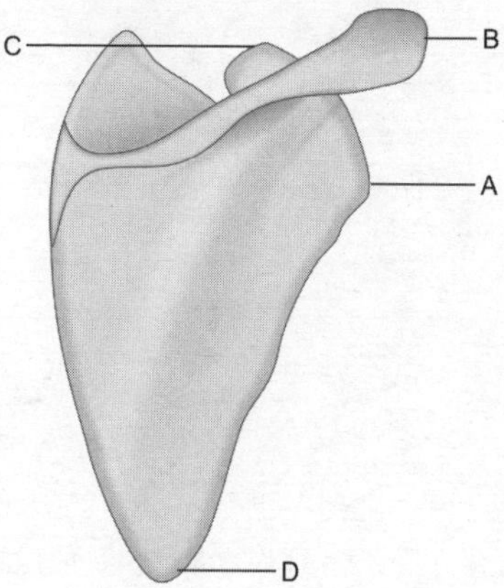

a. A
b. B
c. C
d. D

3. **From which of the following does nucleus pulposus is formed?**

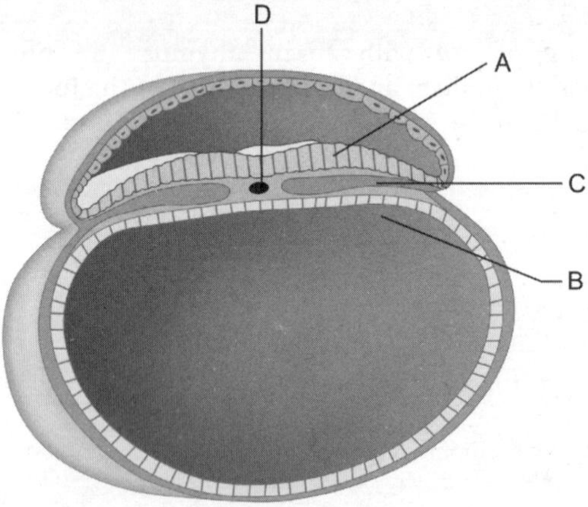

a. A
b. B
c. C
d. D

4. **Through which of the foramen mandibular division of trigeminal nerve passes through?**

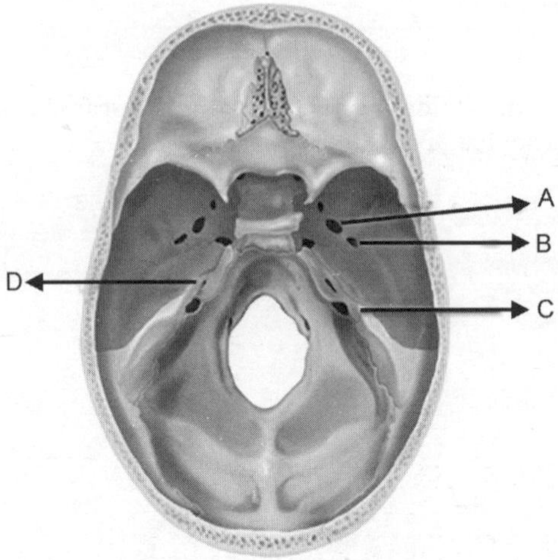

a. A
b. B
c. C
d. D

5. **Which of the following disease pathogenesis primarily involves the marked structure?**

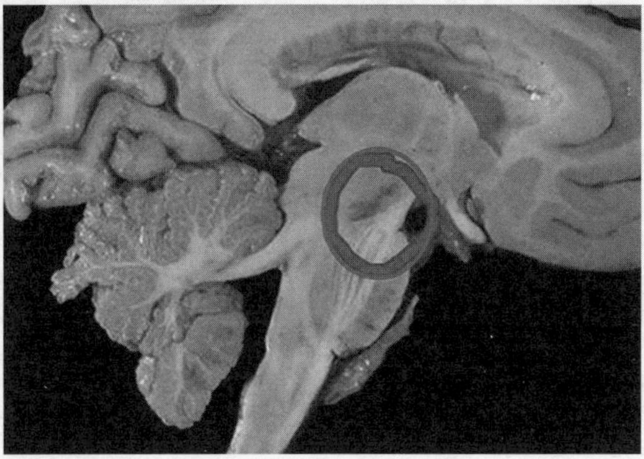

a. Depression
b. Alzheimer's
c. Paralysis agitans
d. Huntington chorea

6. **An arrow pointing to medial rectus muscle. Name the location of the nucleus supplying the muscle?**

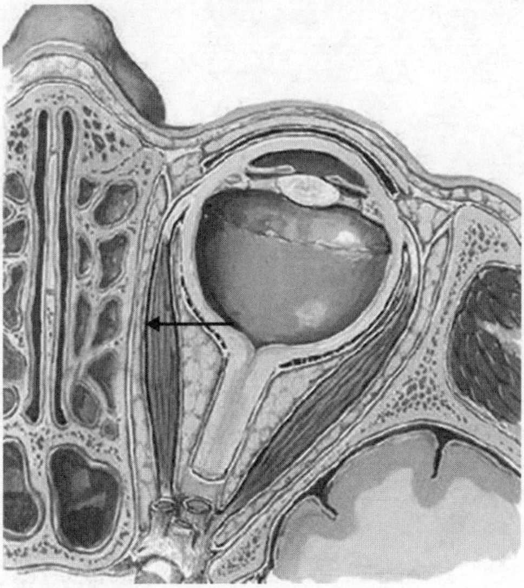

(See Color Plate 1)

a. Facial colliculus
b. Superior colliculus
c. Superior olivary
d. Inferior colliculus

7. **Vertebral artery is related to which of the following areas?**

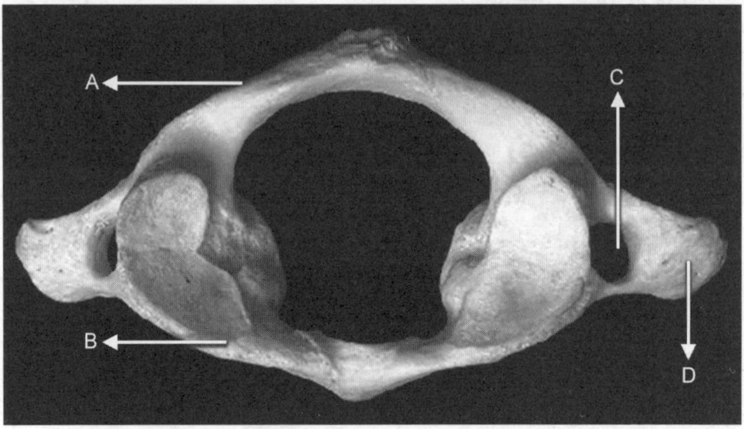

(See Color Plate 1)

a. A
b. B
c. C
d. D

8. **Which of the following is the function of the marked muscles?**

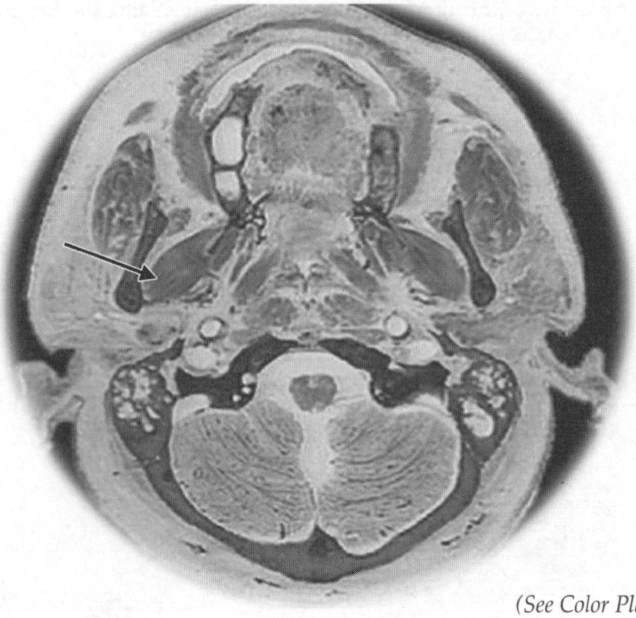

(See Color Plate 1)

a. Protrusion
b. Retrusion
c. Depression
d. Elevation

9. **Which of the following is the origin of the marked fibers?**

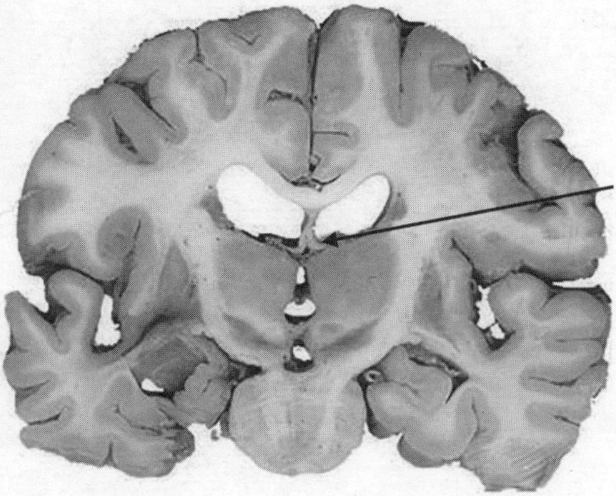

(See Color Plate 2)

a. Mammillary body
b. Hippocampus
c. Habenular
d. Amygdala

10. **The diagram below shows the epiploic foramen. Along the superior boundary the structure marked in the figure corresponds to:**

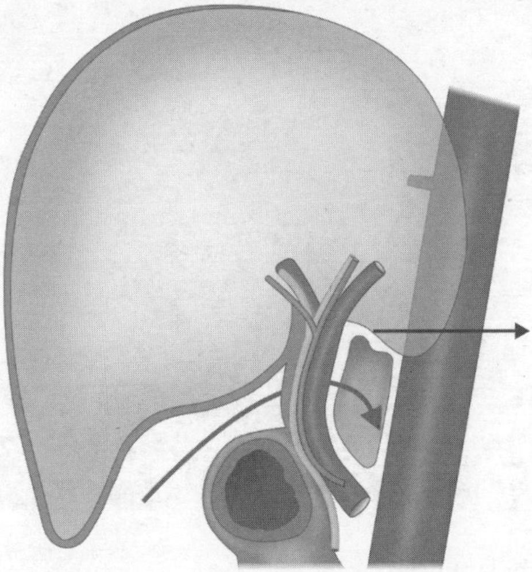

(See Color Plate 2)

a. Lesser omentum
b. Caudate lobe
c. Duodenum
d. IVC

11. **Identify the pelvic diaphragm in the image:**

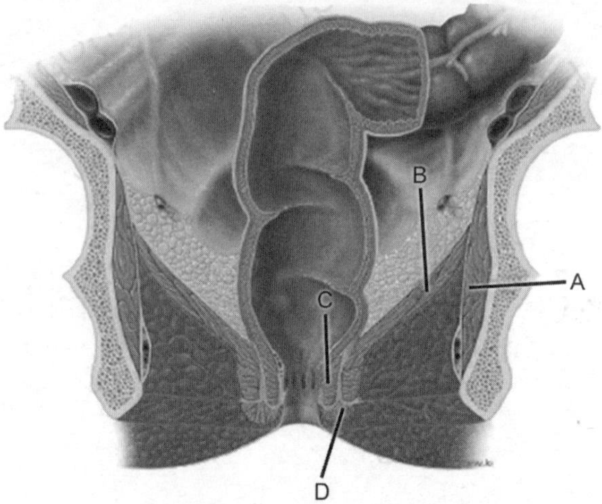

(See Color Plate 2)

a. A　　b. B
c. C　　d. D

12. **The following cell is inhibitory to:**

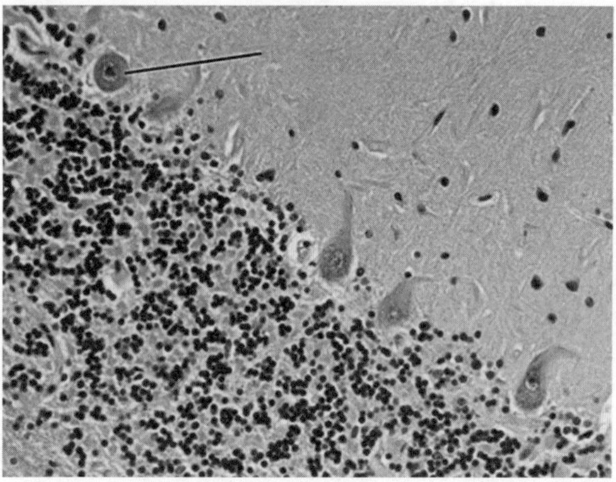

(See Color Plate 3)

a. Vestibular nuclei
b. Deep nuclei of cerebellum
c. Anterior horn of spinal
d. Basal ganglia

13. Below is the insertion of transverse abdominis muscle. Which of the following marks the conjoint tendon?

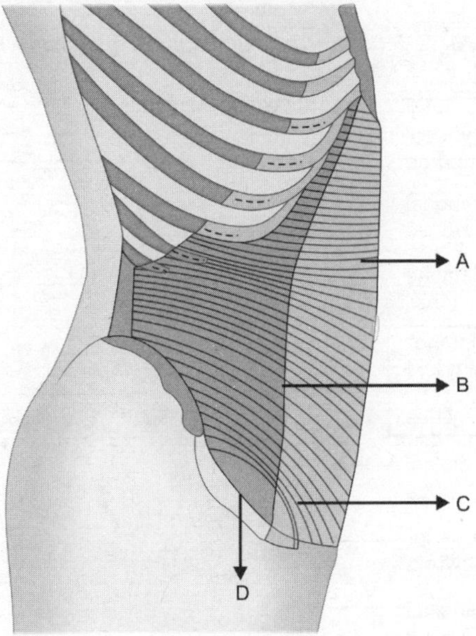

(See Color Plate 3)

a. A
b. B
c. C
d. D

EXPLANATIONS

1. **Ans. a. (A)** *(Ref: Larsen's Human Embryology, p463)*

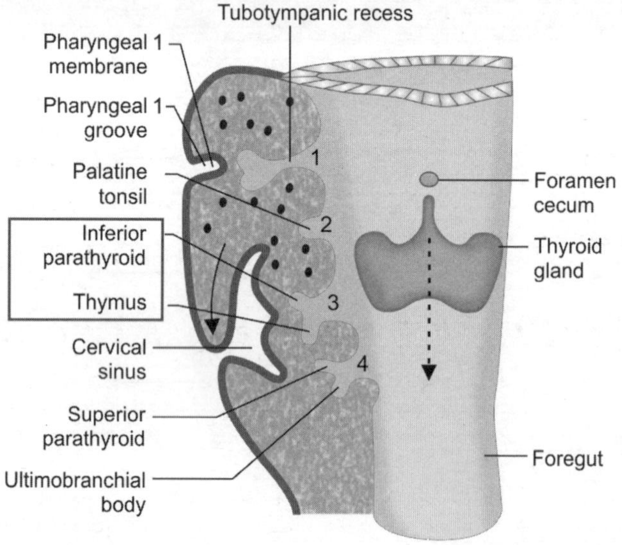

(See Color Plate 3)

1. **Pharyngeal pouch 1:** Develops into the **auditory tube** and **middle ear cavity**
2. **Pharyngeal pouch 2:** Forms numerous infoldings that become the **crypts of the palatine tonsil**; later, lymphocytes (from the thymus and bone marrow) infiltrate the underlying lamina propria to establish the definitive **palatine tonsil**.
3. **Pharyngeal pouch 3:** Divides into a superior (or dorsal) and inferior (or ventral) portion:
   - **Dorsal portion of pouch 3**: Forms the **inferior parathyroid glands**—the chief (or principal) and oxyphil cells are derived from the endodermal lining of the pouch.
   - **Ventral portion of pouch 3:** Forms the **thymus**—the epithelial reticular cells (including those that comprise the thymic or Hassall's corpuscles) are derived from the endodermal lining of the pouch. T-cell progenitors from the bone marrow infiltrate the cortex to establish the definitive thymus.
4. **Pharyngeal pouch 4:** Also divides into a superior (or dorsal) and inferior (or ventral) portion:

- **Dorsal portion of pouch 4:** Forms the **superior parathyroid glands**—the chief (or principal) and oxyphil cells are derived from the endodermal lining of the pouch.
- **Ventral portion of pouch 4:** Forms a diverticulum called the **ultimobranchial body**, the cells of which migrate into the thyroid gland and differentiate into **parafollicular (C) cells of the thyroid gland**.

2. **Ans. c. (C)** *(Ref: Snell's Clinical Anatomy, p425)*

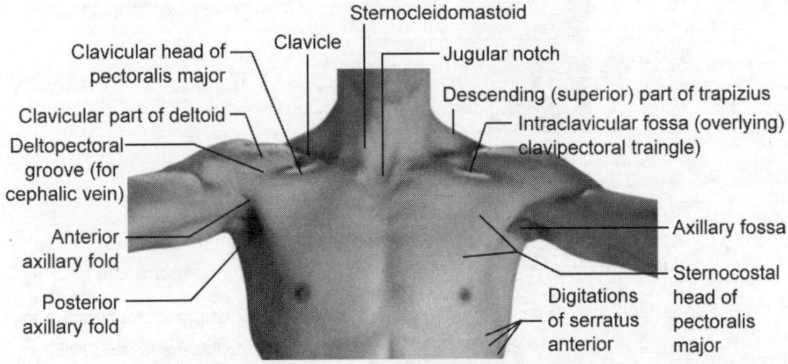

- **Coracoid process:** Palpate under the lateral part of the clavicle (about one inch below the anterior edge of the clavicle).
- **Acromion process:** The lateral end of the spine is free and forms the acromion, which articulates with the clavicle.
- The superolateral angle of the scapula forms the pear-shaped glenoid cavity, or fossa, which articulates with the head of the humerus at the shoulder joint.
- The inferior angle of the scapula can be palpated easily in the living subject and marks the level of the 7th rib and the spine of the 7th thoracic vertebra.

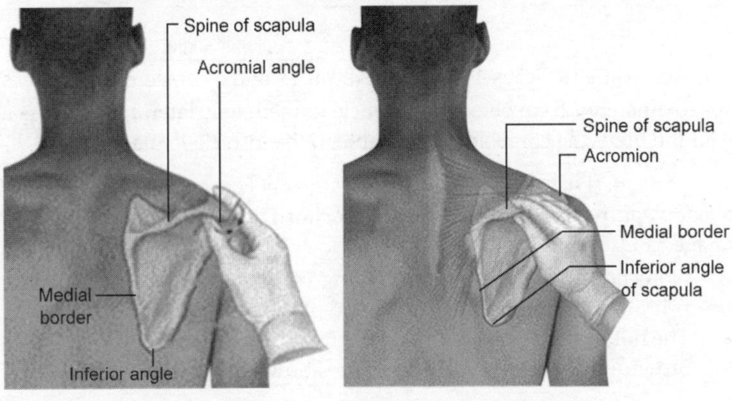

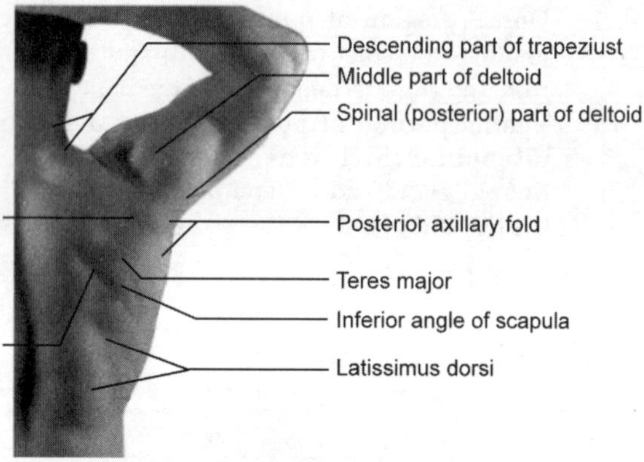

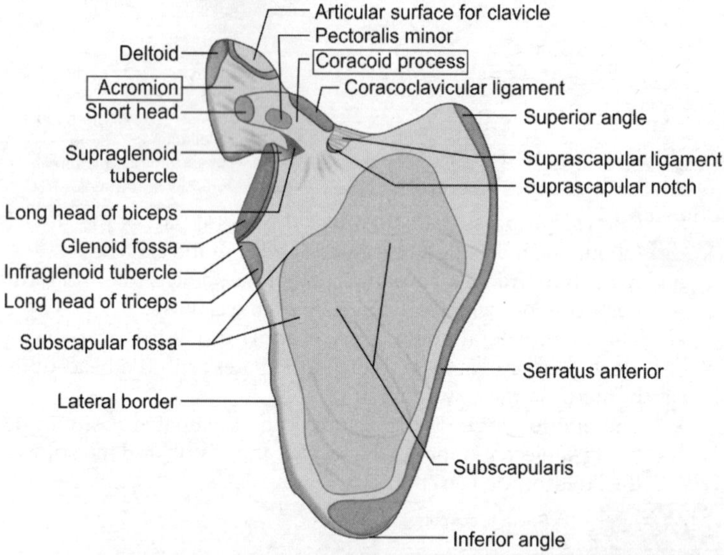

According to Grays 41st edition the apex of the coracoid process lies approximately 2.5 cm below the clavicle immediately lateral to this fossa. And the tip of the coracoids is palpable in the infraclavicular fossa.

3. Ans. d. (D) *(Ref: Essentials of Human Embryology, p258)*

Nucleus pulposus is formed from notochord which has been shown in image as D

- Notochord develops in region lying between the cranial end of the primitive streak and the caudal end of the prochordal plate.
- The notochordal process develops from Notochord.
- Structural changes of notochord are shown in the below diagram.

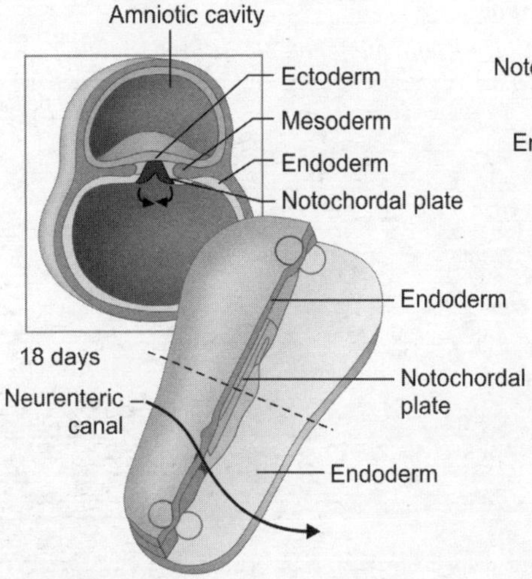

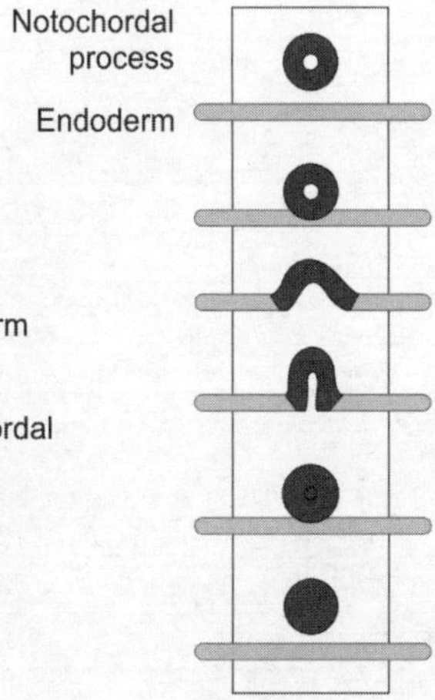

4. Ans. a. (A) *(Ref: Snell's Clinical Anatomy, p676)*

Mandibular division of trigeminal nerve passes through foramen ovale; which is situated in between foramen rotundum and foramen spinosum

Foramen	Structures passing through foramen
Foramen ovale	M: **M**andibular nerve A: **A**ccessory meningeal artery L: **L**esser petrosal nerve E: **E**missary vein
Foramen spinosum	

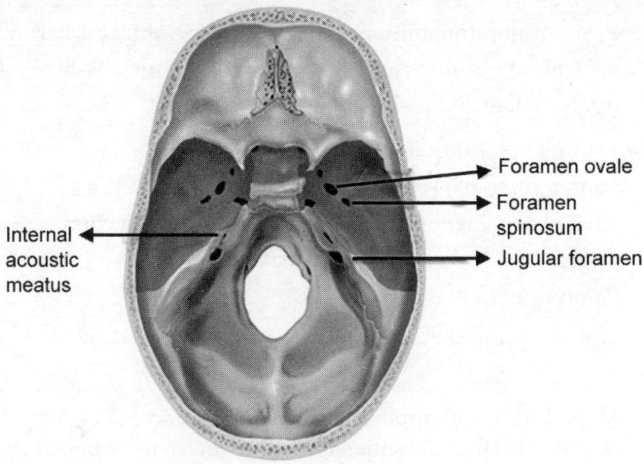

5. **Ans. c. Paralysis agitans**

(Ref: Textbook of Clinical Neuroanatomy, 2/e Vishram Singh, p83, 84)

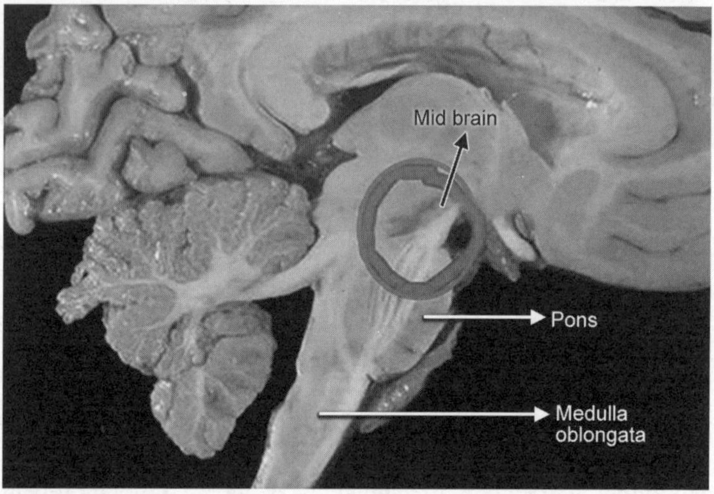

Substantia nigra

- Divided into the posterior (pars compacta) containing large pigmented (melanin) cells and the anterior (pars reticularis).
- Receives gamma—Aminobutyric acid-ergic (GABA-ergic) input from the caudatoputamen (striatonigral fibers).
- Projects dopaminergic fibers to the caudatoputamen (nigrostriatal fibers).
- Projects nondopaminergic fibers to the ventral anterior nucleus, ventral lateral nucleus, and mediodorsal nucleus of the thalamus (nigrothalamic fibers).

Dopamine-containing neurons

- Found in the pars compacta of the substantia nigra.
- Give rise to the dopaminergic nigrostriatal projection.
- Degenerate in Parkinson's disease. This disease is also known as Paralytic agitans.

6. **Ans. b. Superior colliculus**

(Ref: Gray's Anatomy 42/e, p312)

- Medial rectus is supplied by oculomotor nerve [III CN]
- Nucleus of III CN is situated at the level of superior colliculus.

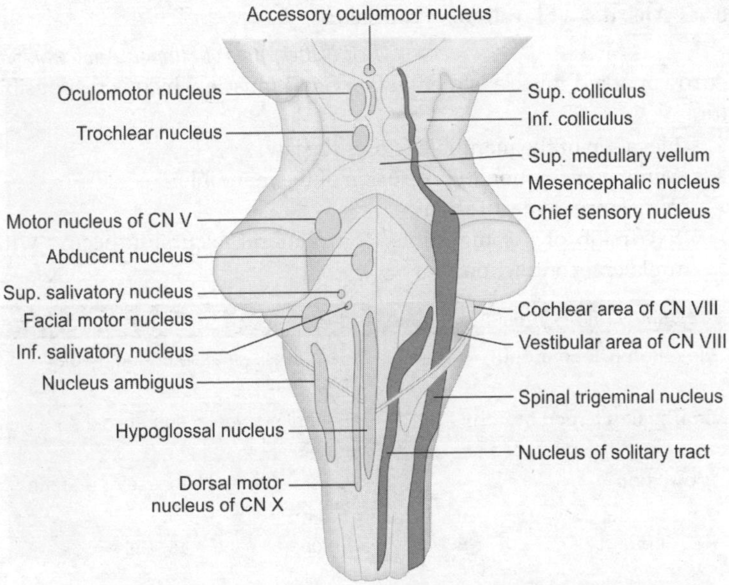

7. **Ans. a. (A)** *(Ref: Gray's Anatomy 41/e, p2830)*

The given diagram is atlas vertebra (superior view) and marker A shows the groove on the posterior arch of atlas, which is related to the third part of vertebral artery.

- **Marker A:** Anterior arch
- **Marker B:** Superior articular facet
- **Marker C: Foramina transversarium**

Vertebral artery passes through foramina transversarium indicated as c in image.

5 branches of vertebral artery:

- Anterior spinal artery
- Posterior spinal artery
- Medullary artery
- Meningeal artery
- Posterior inferior cerebellar artery (PICA)

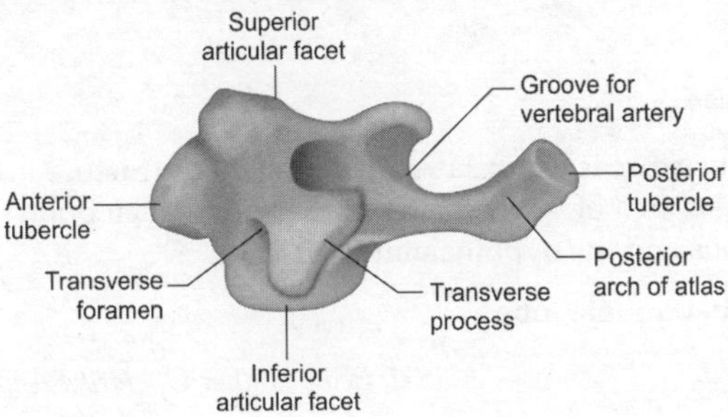

8. Ans. d. > a Elevation > Protrusion

(Ref: Netter Atlas of Human Anatomy, 5/e)

Arrow marked muscle is medial Pterygoid muscle which is responsible for:

- Elevation of the mandible (closes the jaw)
- Minor contribution to protrusion of the mandible
- Assistance in mastication
- Excursion of the mandible; contralateral excursion occurs with unilateral contraction.

Movements of Mandible	Muscle(s)
Elevation (Close mouth)	Temporalis, masseter and medial pterygoid
Depression (Open mouth)	Lateral pterygoid, suprahyoid and infrahyoid
Protrusion	Lateral pterygoid, masseter and medial pterygoid
Retrusion	Temporalis and masseter

9. Ans. b. Hippocampus

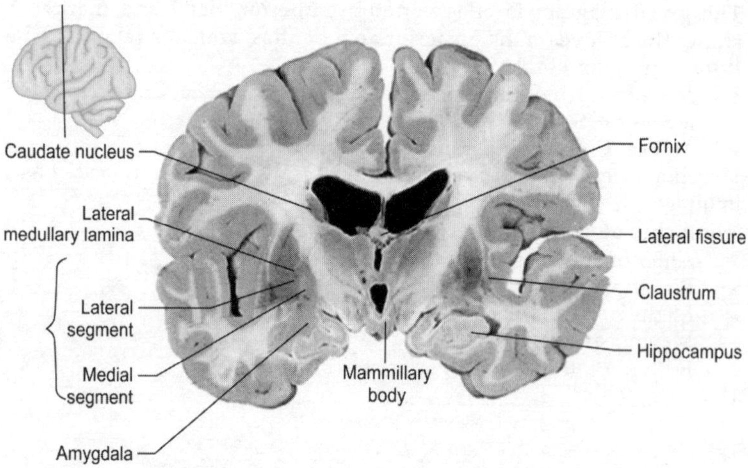

Indicated structure is fornix, a vaulted or arched structure in the body. It is a triangular area of white matter in the mammalian brain between the hippocampus and the hypothalamus.

10. Ans. b. Caudate lobe

(Ref: Scott Conner Operative Anatomy, p479)

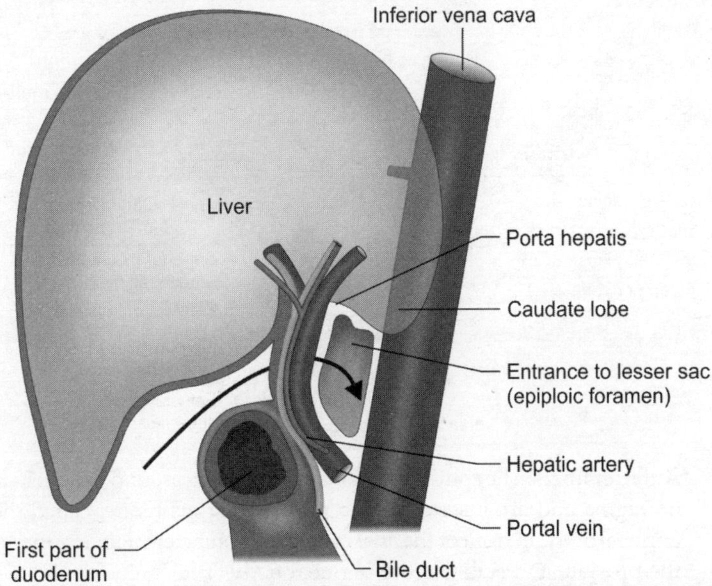

The lesser sac lies behind the stomach and the lesser Omentum. It extends upward as far as the diaphragm and downward between the layers of the greater omentum. The Left margin of the sac is formed by the spleen, gastro splenic ligament and phrenico splenic ligament. The right margin opens into the greater sac (the main part of the peritoneal cavity) through the opening of the lesser sac, or epiploic foramen. The opening into the lesser sac (epiploic foramen) has the following boundaries:

- **Anteriorly:** Free border of the lesser omentum, the bile duct, the hepatic artery, and the portal vein.
- **Posteriorly:** Inferior vena cava
- **Superiorly:** Caudate process of the caudate lobe of the liver
- **Inferiorly:** First part of the duodenum.

11. Ans. b. (B)

(Ref: Cunninghm Anatomy. p456)

Levator ani Muscle

The levator ani muscle is a wide thin sheet that has a linear origin from the back of the body of the pubis, a tendinous arch formed by a thickening of the fascia covering the obturator internus, and the spine of the ischium. From this extensive origin, groups of fibers sweep downward and medially to their insertion as follows:

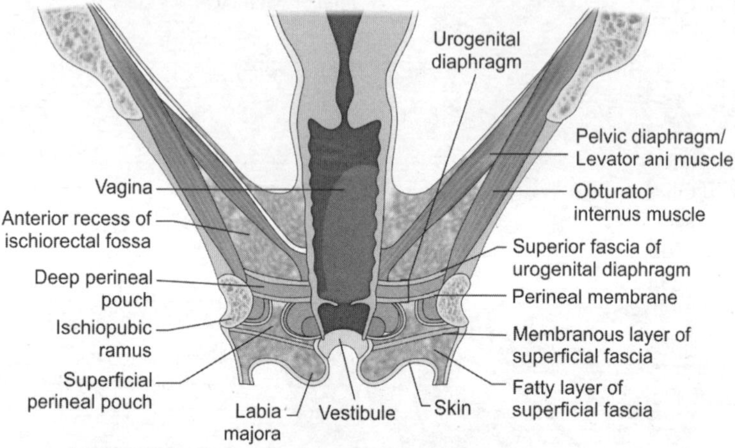

- **Anterior fibers:** The sphincter vaginae form a sling around the prostate or vagina and are inserted into a mass of fibrous tissue, called the perineal body, in front of the anal canal. The sphincter vaginae support the prostate and stabilize the perineal body. The sphincter vaginae constrict the vagina and stabilize the perineal body.
- **Intermediate fibers:** The Puborectalis forms a sling around the junction of the rectum and anal canal. The pubococcygeus passes posteriorly to be inserted into a small fibrous mass, called the anococcygeal body, between the tip of the coccyx and the anal canal.
- **Posterior fibers:** The iliococcygeus is inserted into the anococcygeal body and the coccyx.

12. Ans. b. Deep nuclei of cerebellum

(Ref: Snell Clinical Anatomy. p398)

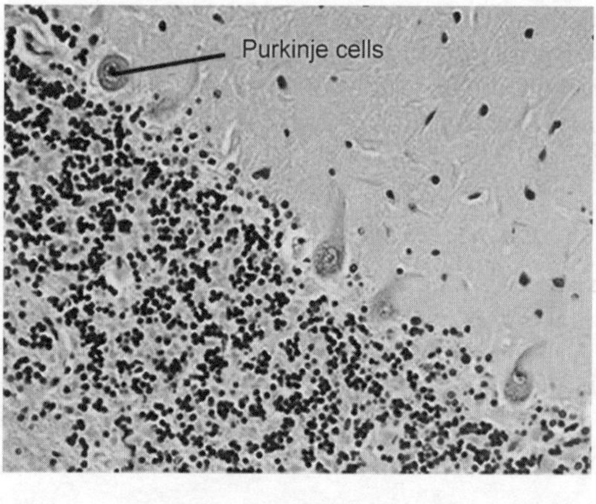

1. Cerebellum is divided into gray and white matter
2. Gray matter is having 3 layers (MP-G):
   - Molecular layer
   - Purkinje layer
   - Granular layer

Excitatory input to Purkinje fibers:

- Olives (directly) (via climbing fibers)
- Mossy fibers (indirectly via granule cell via parallel fibers).

Inhibitory input to Purkinje fibers (and on to parallel fibers):

- Golgi cells
- Stellate cells
- Basket cells.

Purkinje have a net inhibitory output onto deep cerebellar nuclei (which are excitatory).

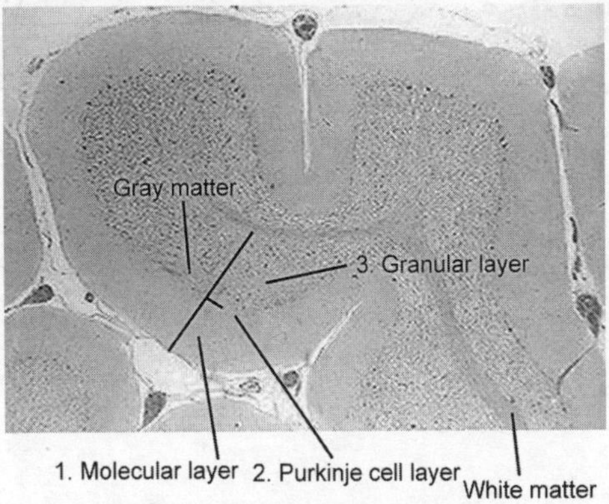

13. Ans. c. (C) *(Ref: Illustrated Anatomy, Kevin Patton, p76)*

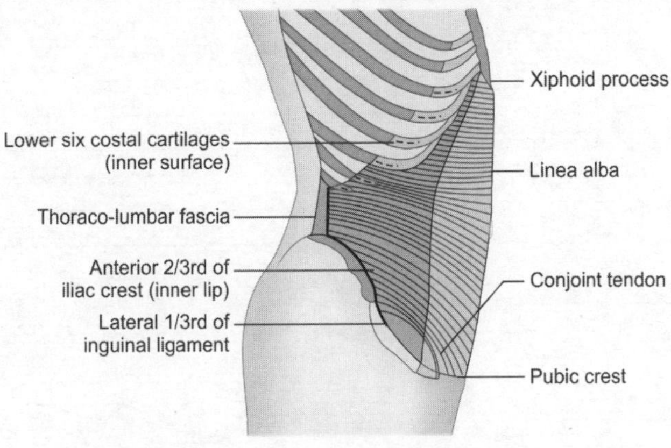

The **conjoint tendon** forms when the medial fibers of the internal oblique aponeurosis unite with the deeper fibers of the transversus abdominis aponeurosis. The conjoint tendon then turns inferiorly and attaches onto the pubic crest and pecten pubis. It forms part of the posterior wall of the inguinal canal.

PHYSIOLOGY

QUESTIONS

1. **Which of the following is the constituent of the marked area in the electron microscopic image of muscle?**

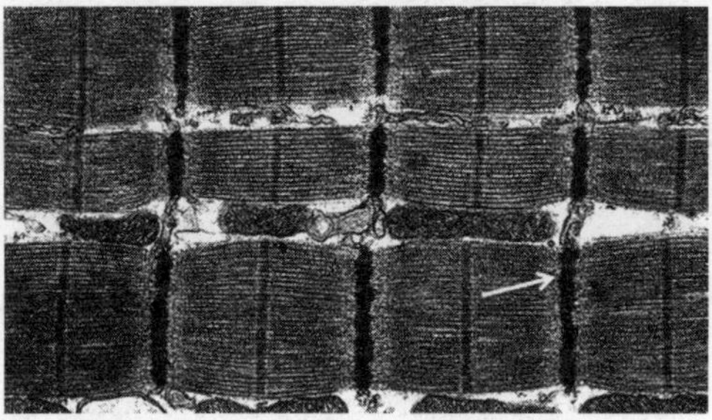

a. Alpha actinin b. Nebulin
c. Titin d. Tropomodulin

2. **Identify the tetanizing frequency of the below demonstration of the gastrocnemius muscle of the frog:**

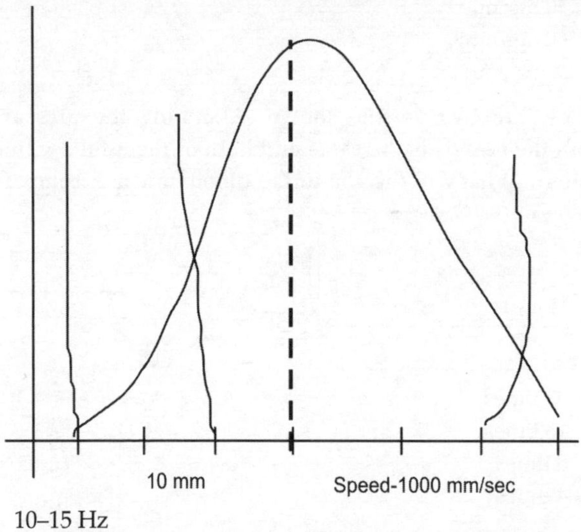

a. 10–15 Hz
b. 15–20 Hz
c. 20–25 Hz
d. 30–35 Hz

3. **A patient with blood glucose level of 200 and GFR of 90. The transport maximum of the patient is as shown in the picture given below. What is the amount of glucose excreted?**

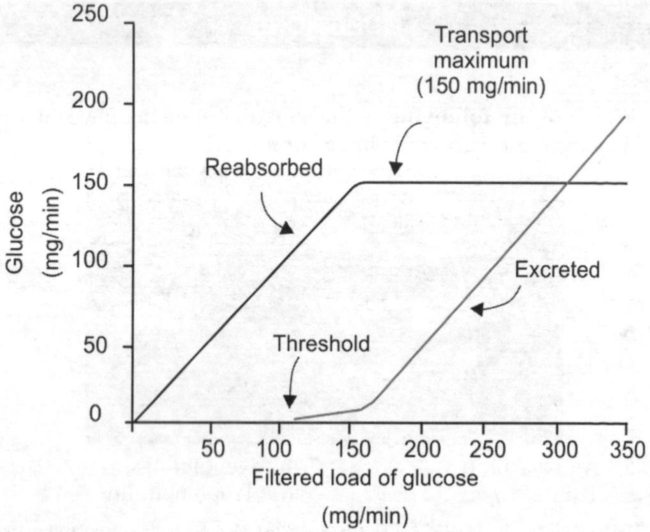

a. 40 mg/min
b. 30 mg/min
c. 60 mg/min
d. 80 mg/min

4. **Below are two vessels shown. Assuming the pressure along both the vessels is the same and both of them follow linear flow pattern. What will the amount of blood flow in A compared to B?**

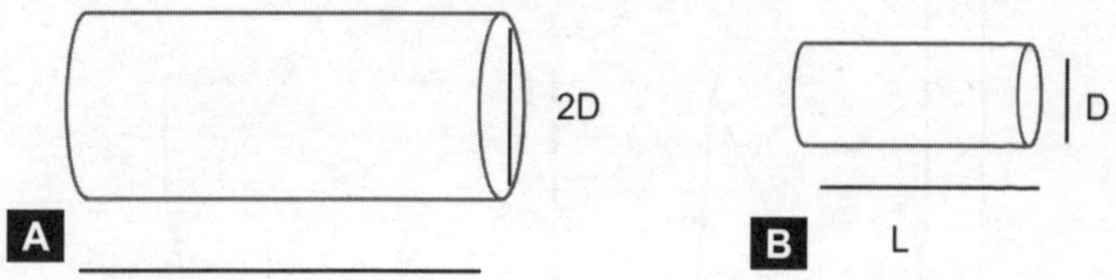

a. 32 times
b. 16 times
c. 8 times
d. 4 times

5. **Below is the picture of phonocardiogram and chest lead ECG. Which of the following marked areas point to the second heart sound?**

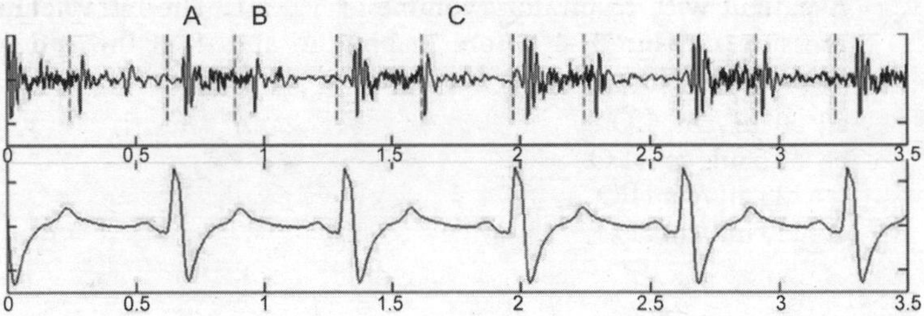

a. A
b. B
c. Not adequate information provided
d. C

6. **The oxygen carrying capacity of an 18-year-old boy with hemoglobin of 14 g/dL is:**
   a. 14
   b. 16
   c. 18
   d. 22

7. **Calculated FEV_1 from the below spirometry reading:**

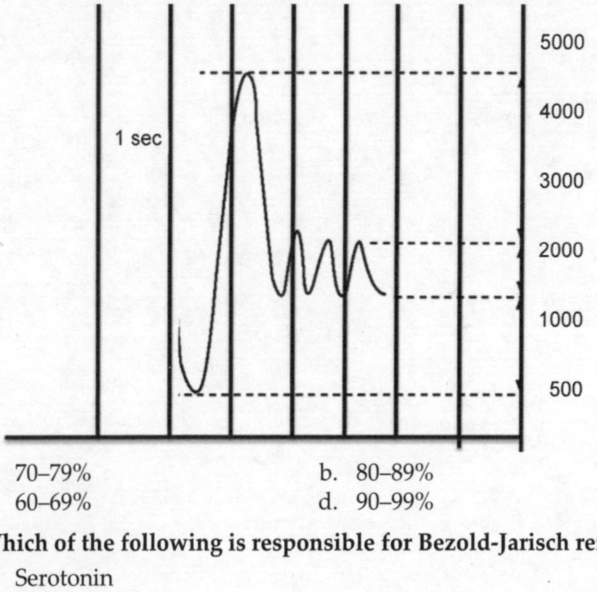

a. 70–79%
b. 80–89%
c. 60–69%
d. 90–99%

8. **Which of the following is responsible for Bezold-Jarisch reflex?**
   a. Serotonin
   b. Histamine
   c. Prostaglandin
   d. Angiotensin

9. A patient with respiratory volume of 500 mL. The intrapleural pressure measured -4 before inspiration and -8 at the end of inspiration. The pulmonary compliance of the patient is:

a. 50 mL/cm H_2O
b. 62.5 mL/cm H_2O
c. 125 mL/cm H_2O
d. 150 mL/cm H_2O

EXPLANATIONS

1. **Ans. a. Alpha actinin** *(Ref: Ganong, 25/e p101)*

Structural proteins in skeletal muscle
Titin: ❍ It is the largest known protein present in mammals ❍ Also called as "muscle spring" because it is responsible for "Elasticity" in muscle ❍ Connects the Z lines to the M lines and provides scaffolding for the sarcomere **Desmin:** ❍ It is the intermediate filament of muscle ❍ It connects Z lines to the plasma membrane **Actinin:** ❍ It binds actin to the Z lines **Dystrophin-Glycoprotein complex:** ❍ Components are dystroglycan, merosin, syntrophins and sarcoglycan.

2. **Ans. d. 30–35 Hz** *(Ref: Ganong, 25/e p107)*

To solve the question:

- Each block corresponds to 10 mm
- Paper speed is 1000 mm/sec
- Contraction period includes 3 blocks. So its 30 mm
- 1000 mm = 1 sec
- 30 mm = 30/1000 = 30 msec
- **So, contraction period** = 30 msec
- **Tetanizing frequency** = 1/contraction period = 1000/30 = 33 Hz

3. **Ans. b. 30 mg/min** *(Ref: Ganong, 25/e p681)*

Transport Maximum:

- In the adult human, the transport maximum for glucose averages about 375 mg/min, whereas the filtered load of glucose is only about 125 mg/min (GFR × plasma glucose = 125 mL/min × 1 mg/mL).
- With large increases in GFR and/or plasma glucose concentration that increase the filtered load of glucose above 375 mg/min, the excess glucose filtered is not reabsorbed and passes into the urine.

Substance	Transport Maximum
Glucose	375 mg/min
Phosphate	0.10 mm/min
Sulfate	0.06 mm/min
Amino acids	1.5 mm/min

Substance	Transport Maximum
Urate	15 mg/min
Lactate	75 mg/min
Plasma protein	30 mg/min
Transport maximums	For substances that are actively secreted also
Substances Exhibit transport maximums as follows:	
Substance	Transport maximum
Creatinine	16 mg/min
Para-aminohippuric acid	80 mg/min

Solving the problem

- **Filtration load**
  GFR × plasma glucose level (in mg/mL)
  = 90 × 2
  = 180
- **T_{max} – in this image it is 150.**
- **Excretion of glucose** = Filtration – Absorption
  = 180–150 = 30 mg/min

4. Ans. c. 8 times *(Ref: Ganong, 25/e p573)*

- Blood flow (F) inside vessel depends on:
  i. Pressure difference (P_A–P_B) – directly related
  ii. Viscosity of the fluid (η) – inversely related
    - Viscosity is the measure of a fluid's resistance to flow.
    - A fluid with low viscosity flows easily. Such fluids are called **Newtonian fluid.** Example is water.
    - A fluid with high viscosity flows resists motion. Such fluids are called Non-Newtonian fluid. Example is blood.
- **Fahraeus-Lindqvist effect –** This effect is seen mainly in capillaries where RBCs flow in the center which leaves cell free plasma near the vessel wall. So, the viscosity change per unit change in hematocrit is much less in capillaries.
  i. Radius of the vessel (r^4) – directly related
  ii. Length of the vessel (L) – inversely related
- Interrelation of these factors are expressed in **Poiseuille-Hagen formula** which is,

$$F = (P_A - P_B) * \pi r^4 / 8 \eta L$$

  - Since, length is doubled and diameter is doubled in vessel A, its flow will be,

$$F = 2^4/2 = 16/2 = 8 \text{ times}$$

5. Ans. b. B *(Ref: Ganong, 25/e p542)*

Phonocardiogram:

- It allows the detection of subaudible sounds and murmurs, and makes a permanent record of these events
- In contrast, the stethoscope cannot always detect all such sounds or murmurs, and it provides no record of their occurrence.

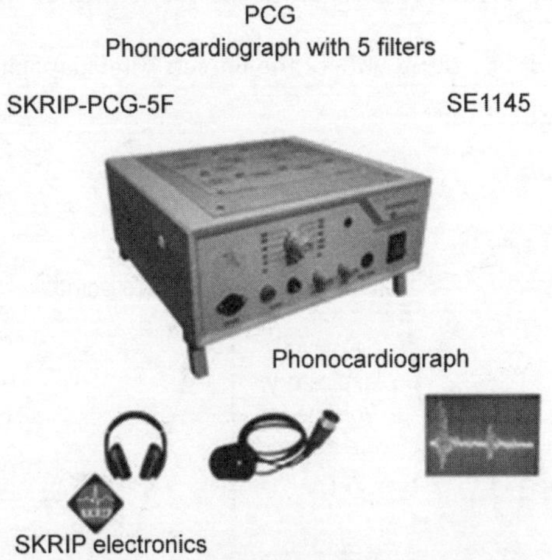

S1	Peak of R wave
S2	End of T wave
S3	Rapid filling phase
S4	End of P wave

6. Ans. c. 18 *(Ref: Ganong, 25/e p640)*

Oxygen carrying capacity of blood:

The theoretical maximum oxygen carrying capacity is 1.39 mL O_2/g Hb, but direct measurement gives a capacity of 1.34 mL O_2/g Hb.

CaO_2 or "Oxygen Content" gives a definite amount of ALL the oxygen in the blood. It is the only method that takes into account how much hemoglobin is actually present in the body and uses the PaO_2 and SaO_2 values to get the amount of oxygen. It uses the units "mL O_2/dL" (milliliters of oxygen per deciliter of blood). CaO_2 is calculated the following way:

CaO_2 = Hb (gm/dL) × 1.34 mL O_2/gm Hb × SaO_2 + PaO_2 × (0.003 mL O_2/mmHg/dL)

Notes: 1.34 mL O_2 is the amount of oxygen that can be bound to 1 g of hemoglobin **0.003 mL O_2** is the amount of oxygen that dissolves in 1 deciliter (dL) of blood.

Oxygen carrying capacity of Hemoglobin

- Each gram of hemoglobin transport 1.34 mL of oxygen
- So, here in the question, its 14 × 1.34 = 18

7. **Ans. b. 80–89%** *(Ref: Ganong, 25/e p630)*

Forced Expiratory Volume in the 1st Second (FEV_1)

- Volume of air that is exhaled in the 1st second of the Forced Vital Capacity
- Normally it is around 80% of the Forced Vital Capacity

Here, in this question:

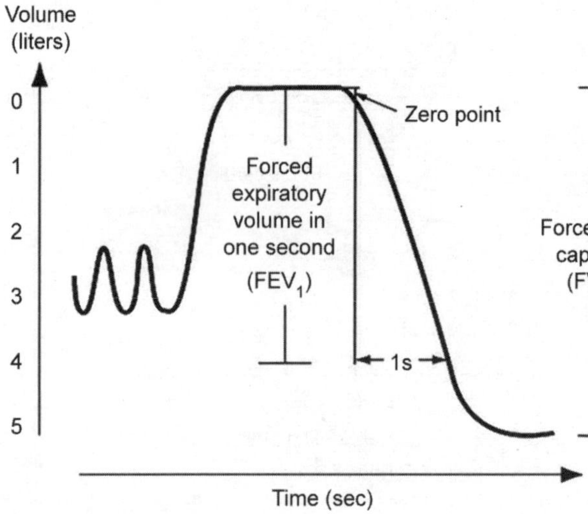

- Forced Vital Capacity = 5L
- FEV_1 = 4L
- So, FEV_1 = 4/5 = 80% of Forced Vital Capacity

A decrease in diffusion capacity (DLCO) indicates interstitial lung disease.

- Forced Expiratory Flow (FEF) 25%–75% primarily reflects the status of the small airways and is more sensitive than the FEV_1 for identifying early airway obstruction.
- It is impaired in bronchiolitis obliterans, smokers, and in patients with lung and heart transplant. Functional residual capacity is measured at the end point of respiration. Functional residual capacity is raised due to increased air trapping in bronchiectasis.
- Residual Volume is equal to Total Lung Capacity minus Vital Capacity.
- Residual Volume is usually 20% of the TLC.

Restrictive lung disorders are characterized by reduced FEV_1 and Forced Vital Capacity, $FEV_1/FVC > 70\%$, reduced TLC and RV and reduced TLCO.

Causes of restrictive lung defect are:

- Neurogenic or psychogenic causes
- Abnormalities of the thoracic wall
- Stiff parenchyma (pulmonary fibrosis)
- Loss of lung tissue, e.g. pneumonectomy
- Displacement

Obstructive lung disorders are characterized by reduced FEV_1 and FVC, $FEV_1/FVC < 70\%$, raised TLC and RV (gas trapping) and reduced TLCO (emphysema) or normal or raised TLCO (asthmatics).

8. **Ans. a. Serotonin** *(Ref: Ganong, 25/e p592, 662)*

Bezold-Jarisch reflex

- Intracardiac injections of chemicals like serotonin, veratridine, capsaicin, phenyldiguanide activates this reflex.
- Afferents for this reflex travel through unmyelinated vagal C fiber endings.
- Clinical importance of **Bezold-Jarisch reflex:**
  - This reflex is responsible for sinus bradycardia seen during myocardial infarction
  - This reflex is one of the cause for profound bradycardia and circulatory collapse after spinal anesthesia.

9. **Ans. b. 62.5 mL/cm H_2O** *(Ref: Guyton, 12/e p467)*

Compliance

- The slope of the pressure-volume curve at a particular lung volume → i.e. volume change per unit of pressure change (mL/cm H_2O)
- Normal value of compliance of intact lung = 200 mLs/cm H_2O
- Lower compliance = more effort of breathing

Specific compliance

- Normal value = 0.05/cm H_2O
- Similar values in both sexes and all ages including neonates
- Is a measurement of the intrinsic elastic property of the lung tissue.

Dynamic compliance vs static compliance

- Static compliance is the compliance measured when there is no gas flow into or out of the lung

Lung compliance and chest wall compliance

- Compliance is made up of lung compliance and chest compliance --> $1/Ct = 1/Cl + 1/Ccw$
  - * i.e. Summation of elastance (= 1/compliance)

- Thus, $1/Ct = 1/200 + 1/200$
- $\rightarrow Ct = 100$ mLs/cm H_2O

NB:

- Ct = total compliance
- Cl = lung compliance
- Cw = chest wall compliance

Compliance is defined as ability of lungs and pleural cavity to change in volume based on pressure changes.

Definition: $\mathbf{C = \Delta V / \Delta P}$

- Compliance is change in volume/change in pressure.
  = 500/8 => 62.5 mL/cm H_2O

BIOCHEMISTRY

QUESTIONS

1. **Which of the following is not seen in low insulin-glucagon ratio?**
   a. Gluconeogenesis
   b. Glycogen breakdown
   c. Ketogenesis
   d. Glycogen storage

2. **Which of the following is anaplerotic reaction?**
   a. Conversion of pyruvate to lactic acid
   b. Conversion of pyruvate to oxaloacetate
   c. Conversion of pyruvate to acetyl COA
   d. Conversion of pyruvate to acetaldehyde

3. **Thiamine deficiency results in decrease energy production, because TPP:**
   a. Interferes with alcohol metabolism
   b. Interferes with transketolase activity
   c. Is cofactor for pyruvate and alpha-ketoglutarate dehydrogenase
   d. Interferes with energy production from amino acids

4. **A young lady presented with tingling sensation in legs and hands. On examination she had fissure tongue and lesions in angle of mouth. On investigation, she had low RBC glutathione reductase activity. Diagnosis is deficiency of:**
   a. Vitamin B2
   b. Vitamin B6
   c. Vitamin B12
   d. Vitamin B1

5. **Phenylbutyrate is used in urea cycle disorders because it:**
   a. Scavenges nitrogen
   b. Activates enzymes
   c. Maintains renal output
   d. Maintains energy production

6. **Which of the following yields 3 molecules of ATP under anaerobic metabolism?**
   a. Glucose
   b. Galactose
   c. Glycogen
   d. Amino acid

7. **Thermogenic food is which of the following?**
   a. High protein diet
   b. High carbohydrate diet
   c. High fat diet
   d. It does not depend on the macronutrients

8. **In chronic diabetics the value of TG and VLDL are more because:**
   a. Increased in activity of hepatic lipase
   b. Increase in peripheral function of LDL receptors
   c. Increased activity of lipoprotein lipase and decreased activity of hormone sensitive lipase
   d. Increased activity of hormone sensitive lipase and decreased lipoprotein lipase activity

9. **Restriction Fragment Length Polymorphism (RFLP) was used in-order to identify the five different species of staphylococci in a surgical ICU. Which of the following site does the restriction enzyme act?**
   a. TAGATA – ATCTAT
   b. ATGGAC – TACGTG
   c. AATATA – TATAAT
   d. GATATC – CTATAG

10. **Which of the following is true regarding Mitochondrial DNA?**
    a. One set from each parents
    b. It has 3 × 109 base pairs
    c. It has more mutations than human DNA
    d. It codes for less than 20% of oxidative phosphorylation proteins

EXPLANATIONS

1. Ans. d. Glycogen storage

Low insulin/glucagon ratio → means low insulin levels and high glucagon levels.

Process	Insulin	Glucagon
Gluconeogenesis	Inhibited (inhibition of pyruvate carboxylase, phosphoenolpyruvate carboxykinase, glucose 6 phosphatase)	Increased (inhibition of pyruvate kinase, phosphofructokinase; activation of fructose 1,6-bisphosphatase)
Glycogenolysis	Inhibited (inhibition of glycogen phosphorylase)	Increased (activation of glycogen phosphorylase)
Ketogenesis	Inhibited [less substrate acetyl coenzyme A (CoA); inhibition of 3-hydroxy-3-methylglutaryl-coenzyme A (HMG CoA) synthetase]	

From the above table it is evident that Gluconeogenesis, glycogenolysis and ketogenesis all are activated in low insulin/glucagon ratio (fasting state).

High Yield—Extra Edge

Relationships between hormonal controls, metabolite transport and major metabolic pathways.
❍ **Fed state = glycolysis + lipogenesis** *(dominated by by insulin, leptin, cholecystokinin)*
❍ **Fasted state = lipolysis + gluconeogenesis + ketogenesis** *(dominated by glucagon and corticosteroids)*
❍ **Working state = lipolysis + glycolysis + gluconeogenesis + ketogenesis** *(physical activity, dominated by adrenalin and IL-6)*
❍ **Sleeping state = tissue growth and repair** *(dominated by growth hormone and IGF1)*
❍ **Infected/cachectic state = hypermetabolism; gluconeogenesis + lipolysis + proteolysis** ❍ *(dominated by pro-inflammatory cytokines, TNF-α, IL-1 & IL-6] and corticosteroids)*
❍ **All states: ureogenesis proceeds in a regulated manner to dispose of surplus nitrogen, controlled by unknown mechanisms.**

2. **Ans. b. Conversion of pyruvate to oxaloacetate**

(Ref: DM Vasudevan, Textbook of Biochemistry for Medical Students, 7/e p253)

- **Anaplerotic reactions** are chemical **reactions** that form intermediates of a metabolic pathway
- The TCA cycle is a hub of metabolism, with central importance in both energy production and biosynthesis.
- Therefore, it is crucial for the cell to regulate concentrations of TCA cycle metabolites in the mitochondria.
- Anaplerotic flux must balance cataplerotic flux in order to retain homeostasis of cellular metabolism

From	To	Notes
Pyruvate	Oxaloacetate	This reaction is catalyzed by pyruvate carboxylase, an enzyme activated by acetyl-CoA, indicating a lack of oxaloacetate. It occurs in animal mitochondria. Most important anaplerotic reaction; depending on severity, deficiency causes lactic acidosis, severe psychomotor deficiency or death in infancy. Pyruvate can also be converted to L-malate, another intermediate, in a similar way.
Aspartate	Oxaloacetate	This is a reversible reaction forming oxaloacetate from aspartate in a transamination reaction, via aspartate transaminase.
Glutamate	α-ketoglutarate	This reaction is catalyzed by glutamate-dehydrogenase.
β-Oxidation of fatty acids	Succinyl-CoA	When odd-chain fatty acids are oxidized, one molecule of succinyl-CoA is formed per fatty acid. The final enzyme is methylmalonyl-CoA mutase. Triheptanoin [fat with three heptanoic (C7:0) fatty acids] may be used to treat pyruvate carboxylase deficiency
Adenylo-succinate	Fumarate	This reaction is catalyzed by adenylosuccinate lyase and occurs in purine synthesis and purine nucleotide cycle. Defect of this enzyme causes psychomotor retardation.

3. **Ans. c. Is cofactor for pyruvate and alpha-ketoglutarate dehydrogenase** *(Ref: Harper's Illustrated Biochemistry, 30/e p556)*

Thiamine pyrophosphate (**TPP**) is a derivative of thiamine (vitamin B1). Nutritional deficiency of thiamine leads to the disease **beriberi**.

Beriberi affects especially the brain, because TPP is required for carbohydrate metabolism, and the brain depends on glucose metabolism for energy.

Pyruvate carboxylase complex – Energy Metabolism

Enzyme	Abbreviated	Prosthetic Group
Pyruvate dehydrogenase	E_1	Thiamine pyrophosphate (TPP)
Dihydrolipoyl transacetylase	E_2	Lipoamide
Dihydrolipoyl dehydrogenase	E_3	FAD

Thiamine and Energy metabolism

- The role of thiamine in energy metabolism is obviously that of it's co-enzyme action for the enzyme pyruvate dehydrogenase which is a part of the pyruvate dehydrogenase complex.
- This complex is essential for conversion of pyruvate to acetyl-CoA . Acetyl-CoA is essential for sending the fate of glucose after glycolysis into the Krebs cycle. Krebs cycle has the best efficiency of returning 10 ATPs per cycle for one acetyl CoA.
- So deficiency of TPP would eventually affect this pathway with respect to energy metabolism.

4. **Ans. a. Vitamin B2**

(Ref: Biochemistry Manual, R Harvey, p242)

Cheilitis angular stomatitis are all classical features of riboflavin and hence the answer is Vitamin B2.

RIBOFLAVIN (Vit. B2)

- **A_2 – 2 ATPs (**FAD and **F**MN are derived from ribo**F**lavin**)**
- **B_2** – Vitamin B2
- **C_2** – Riboflavin deficiency
  - Cheilosis (inflammation of lips, angular stomatitis, magenta-colored tongue)
  - Corneal neovascularization

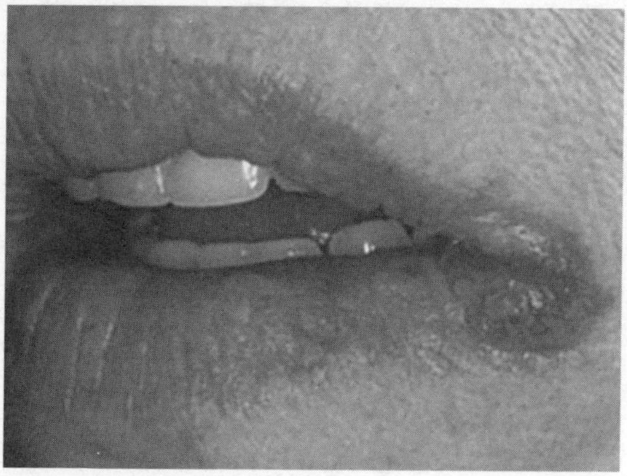

5. Ans. a. Scavenges nitrogen

(Ref: Biochemistry Manual, R. Harvey, p256)

Sodium phenylbutyrate metabolites allows the kidneys to excrete excess nitrogen in place of urea and coupled with dialysis, amino acid supplements and a protein-restricted diet, children born with urea cycle disorders can usually survive beyond 12 months.

Urea cycle – simplified flow chart

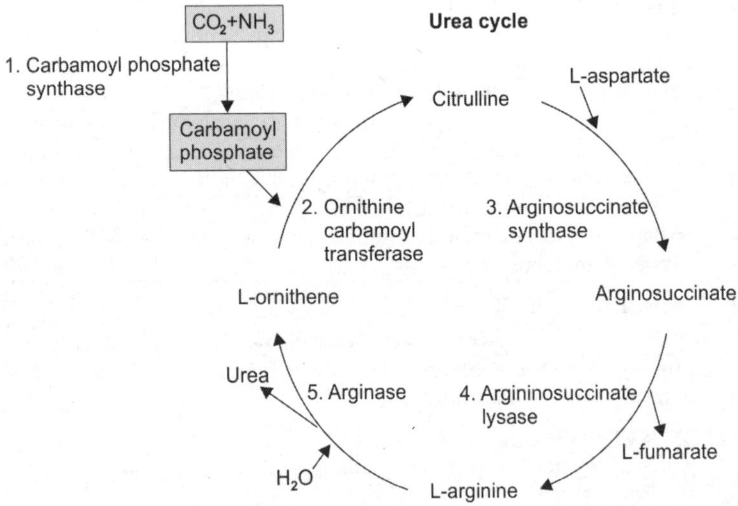

6. Ans. c. Glycogen

(Ref: Textbook of Biochemistry, Richard Harvey, p123)

Glycogen metabolism and energy production

- One molecule of glycogen can yield a massive number of glucose-6 phosphate molecules.
- So technically speaking the net yield of ATPs is large for one molecule of glycogen.
- But if we assume that the question tends to seek the number of ATPs from one glucose molecule extracted from one glycogen molecule then the answer is 3.
- If a free glucose is fermented it yields 2 ATPs.
- But glycogen releases glucose as glucose- 6-phosphate due to the absence of glucose 6-phosphatase.

7. Ans. a. High protein diet

(Ref: Textbook of Biochemistry, Pankaja Naik, p347)

The main determinant of DIT (Diet induced thermogenesis) is the energy content of the food, followed by the **protein fraction of the food.**

- The intestinal absorption of nutrients, the initial steps of their metabolism and the storage of the absorbed but not immediately oxidized nutrient.

Reported DIT values for separate nutrients are:
0 to 3% for fat
5 to 10% for carbohydrate
10 to 30% for alcohol
20 to 30% for protein

- Alcohol energy is largely additive to the normal diet but does not seem to affect energy balance positively. Hence Protein is a better answer to be chosen.

8. **Ans. d. Increased activity of hormone sensitive lipase and decreased lipoprotein lipase activity**

(Ref: Clinical biochemistry, William Marshall, p290)

Lipases and diabetes:

- Lipoprotein lipase has pivotal role in the metabolism of both triglyceride-rich particles and high density lipoproteins.
- Enzyme activity in both adipose tissue and skeletal muscle is insulin dependent, hence varies with DM severity.
- In insulin deficiency/untreated type 1 diabetes, the enzyme activity in both adipose tissue and muscle tissue is low but increases upon insulin therapy.
- In untreated type 2 diabetic patients, the average enzyme activity in adipose tissue and post-heparin plasma is normal or subnormal.
- Therapy with oral agents or insulin, resulting in good glycemic control, is followed by an increase of LPL activity in both adipose tissue and post-heparin plasma.

In both Type 1 and 2 diabetes, changes of Lipoprotein lipase activity are associated with relevant alterations in lipoprotein pattern.

- In insulin deficiency with low LPL, serum total and VLDL triglyceride levels are elevated, and HDL concentration is reduced.
- In chronically insulin-treated patients with high LPL activity, VLDL triglyceride concentrations are normal or subnormal, and HDL level is increased.

Taking into account of the above facts, the most probable answer is D.

9. **Ans. d. GATATC – CTATAG**

(Ref: Textbook of Biochemistry, Pankaja Naik, p465)

Restriction enzyme:

- Restriction enzymes are **DNA-cutting enzymes.**
- A **palindromic sequence** is a sequence made up of nucleic acids within double helix of DNA and/or RNA that is the same when read from 5′ to 3′ on one strand and 5′ to 3′ on the other, complementary strand. It is also known as a palindrome or an inverted-reverse sequence.
- **Restriction enzymes cleave at the palindromic sites.**
- Usually the palindromic sequence will be 4–6 nucleotides length

10. Ans. c. It has more mutations than human DNA

(Ref: Clinical Biochemistry, William Marshall, p468)

Difference between Human and Mitochondrial DNA (each point is important)

Comparison between the human nuclear and mitochondrial genomes*		
Characteristic	**Nuclear genome**	**Mitochondrial genome**
Size	~3.3×10^9 bp	16,569 bp
Number of DNA molecules per cell	23 in haploid cells; 46 in diploid cells	Severa thousand copies per cell (polyploidy)
Number of genes encoded	~20,000–30,000	37 (13 polypepitides, 22 tRNAs and 2 rRNAs)
Gene density	~1 per 40,000 bp	1 per 450 bp
Introns	Frequently found in most genes	Absent
Percentage of coding DNA	~3%	~93%
Codon usage	The universal genetic code	AUA codes for methionine; TGA codes for tryptophan; AGA and AGG specify stop codons
Associated proteins	Nucleosome-associated histone proteins and non-histone proteins	No histones; but associated with several proteins (for example, TFAM) that form nucleoids
Mode of inheritance	Mendelian inheritance for autosomes and the X chromosome; paternal inheritance for the Y chromosome	Exclusively maternal
Replication	Strand-coupled mechanism that uses DNA polymerases α and δ	Strand-coupled and strand-displacement models; only uses DNA polymerase γ

Contd...

Contd...

Characteristic	Nuclear genome	Mitochondrial genome
Transcription	Most genes are transcribed individually	All genes on both strands are transcribed as large polycistrons
Recombination	Each pair of homologous recombines during the prophase of meiosis	There is evidence that recombination occurs at a cellular level but little evidence that it occurs at a population level

PATHOLOGY

QUESTIONS

1. **A 50-year-old male presented with blurring of vision. Urine examination showed proteinuria. Fundus examination showed dot and blot hemorrhages, microaneurysm and cotton wool spots. Histopathology pic of kidney given below. Your diagnosis:**

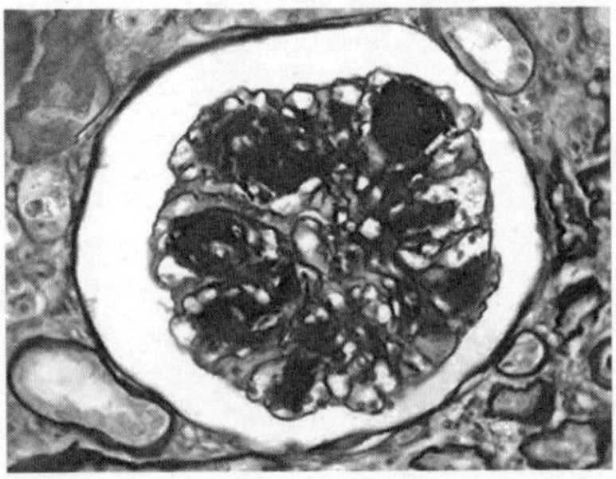

(See Color Plate 4)

   a. Kimmelstiel-Wilson nodules
   b. Crescents
   c. Amyloid
   d. Segmental sclerosis

2. **A 20-year-old female presented with painful blister in skin and oral mucosa. Direct immunofluorescence picture of which is given below. Which of the following is not true regarding the same?**

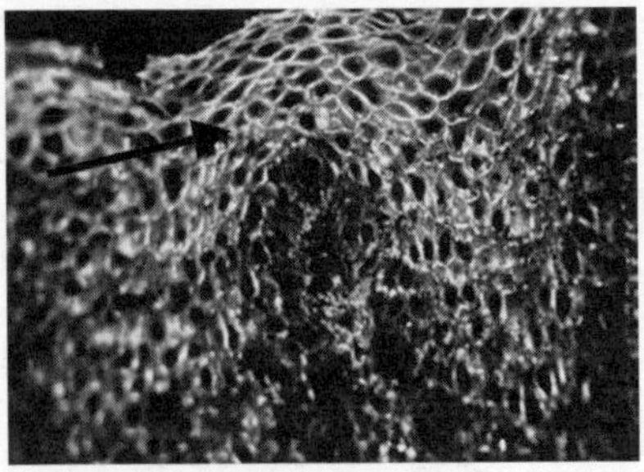

(See Color Plate 4)

   a. Antibodies against hemidesmosomes
   b. Antibodies against desmoglein 1
   c. Antibodies against desmoglein 3
   d. Basement membrane deposition of IgG is the most common DIF picture in bullous lesions

3. **What does the red cell distribution width (RDW) deal with?**
   a. Hypochromia
   b. Anisocytosis
   c. Poikilocytosis
   d. Anisochromia

4. **Which of the following is a negative acute phase reactant?**
   a. Albumin
   b. Haptoglobin
   c. Ferritin
   d. C reactive protein

5. **A 50-year-old male presented with recurrent bloody diarrhea. Colonoscopy showed geographical ulcers. Histopathology is shown below. Your diagnosis:**

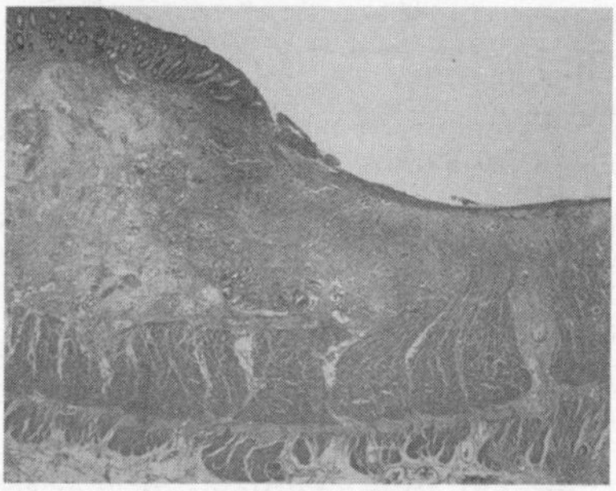

(See Color Plate 4)

   a. Pseudomembranous colitis
   b. Non-Hodgkin lymphoma colon
   c. Adenocarcinoma colon
   d. Crohn's disease

6. **All of the following are seen in the development of T lymphocyte at a point *except*:**
   a. Tdt
   b. CD34
   c. PAX5
   d. Cd1a

7. **Which of the following can change the gene expression by methylation and acetylation without changing content of the gene?**
   a. Translocation
   b. Inversion
   c. Mutation
   d. Epigenetics

8. **If the RB gene phosphorylation is defective which of the following will happen?**
   a. Cell cycle will stop at G2
   b. Cell cycle will stop at G1
   c. There will be no effect on cell cycle as RB gene phosphorylation is not needed
   d. The cell cycle progresses and cell divides

9. **Which of the following plays a role in gene editing?**
   a. Gene Xpert
   b. CRISPR
   c. Health care apps
   d. Big data

10. **Endometriotic lesion histology represents its:**
   a. High estrogen
   b. High insulin
   c. High cholesterol
   d. High levels of prolactin

11. **Which of the following neoplasms shows ALK positivity?**
   a. Ewing sarcoma
   b. Inflammatory myofibroblastic tumor
   c. Synovial sarcoma
   d. Fibromatosis

12. **During development all the antigens of ones self are introduced to thymic cells in-order to be removed to prevent autoimmunity. Which of the following genes is involved in the process?**
   a. NOTCH1
   b. AIRE
   c. RB gene
   d. CPK gene

13. **Which of the following cells have MHC class II?**
   a. RBC
   b. B cells, Dendritic cells, NK cells
   c. All nucleated cells
   d. Platelets

14. **Which of the following Immunohistochemistry marker is used in cyclin D1 negative Mantle cell lymphoma?**
   a. SOX11
   b. ITRA 1
   c. MYD88
   d. Annexin V

15. **A 60-year-old male with complaints for frothy urine and facial puffiness. The DIF and electron microscopic picture of the patient is given below. Diagnosis is:**

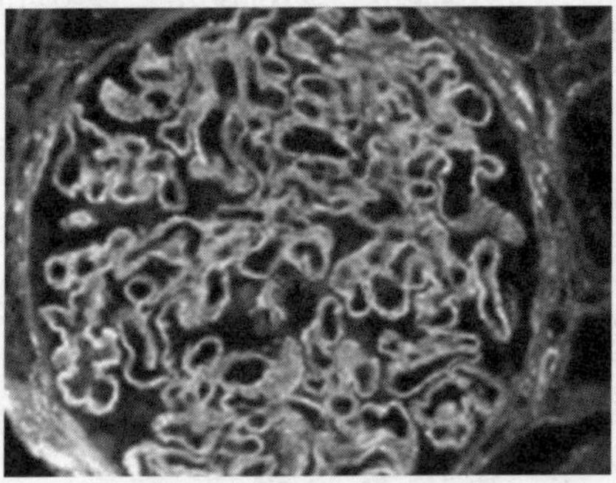

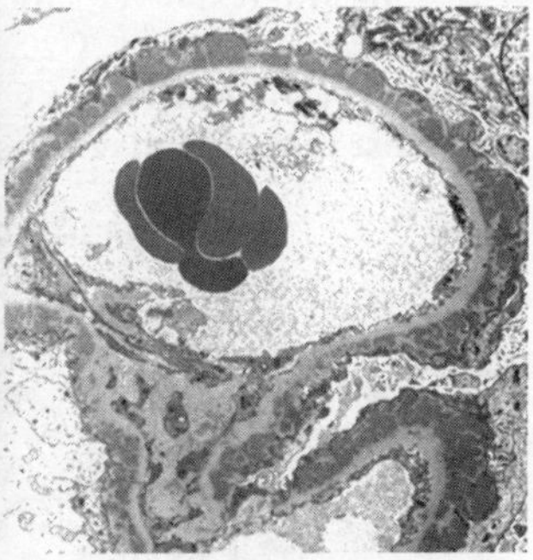

(See Color Plate 5)

a. Membranoproliferative nephritis
b. Membranous glomerulopathy
c. Minimal change disease
d. FSGS

16. **A 7-year-old with fever, weight loss. On examination he was pale and had significant lymphadenopathy. Bone marrow histology of the person is as given below. Your diagnosis is:**

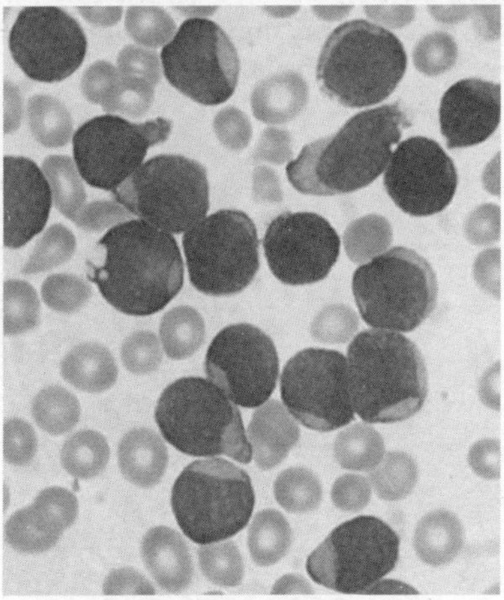

(See Color Plate 5)

a. ALL
b. AML
c. Aplastic anaemia
d. Juvenile myelomonocytic leukemia

17. A 35-year-old presented with fever. On examination he had enlarged and ulcerated tonsils. His peripheral blood smear showed lymphocytosis. Monospot test was negative. Tonsillectomy was done and it showed large cells mixed with lymphocytes. The cells were positive for CD20, EBVLMP1, MUM1, CD 79a. Background cells were positive for CD3. The cells are negative for CD15. Your most probable diagnosis:

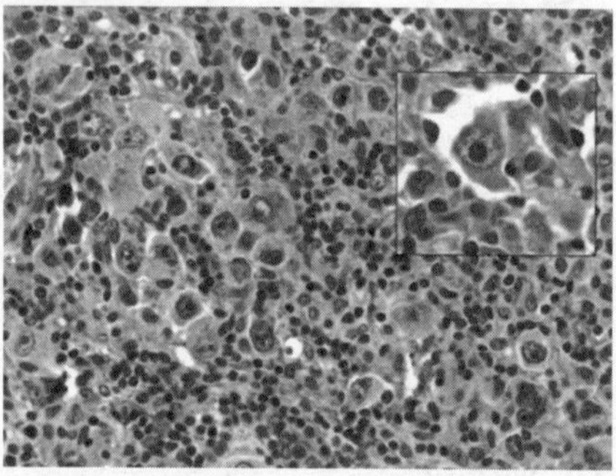

(See Color Plate 5)

a. Infectious mononucleosis
b. Hodgkin lymphoma
c. EBV positive – DLBL
d. EBV positive mucocutaneous ulcer

18. A 40-year-old patient presented with heart burn and increased salivation. UGE scopy was done and biopsy was taken and is as shown below. Which of the is the diagnosis?

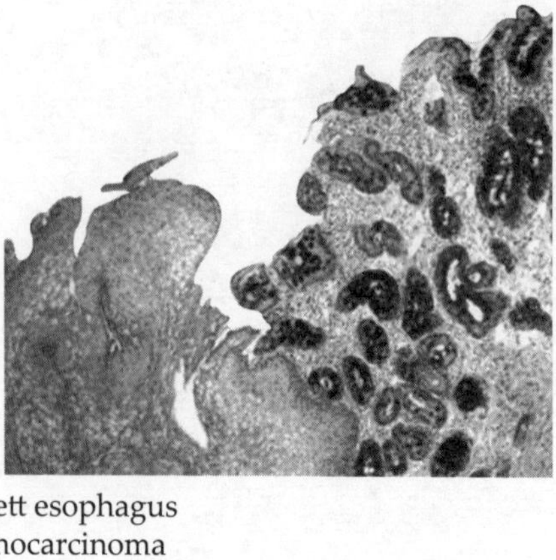

(See Color Plate 6)

a. Barrett esophagus
b. Adenocarcinoma
c. Esophagitis
d. Squamous cell carcinoma

19. A 25-year-old female came to OPD, 1 year after postpartum. She was treated for iron deficiency anemia while pregnancy. Now she was pale and her Hb was 5% and reticulocyte count was 9%. Her corrected retic count is:

a. 6
b. 4.5
c. 3
d. 1

20. Acetone free ethanol in leishman stain does which of the following?

a. Fixes cells to slide
b. Color of cell
c. Causes metabolic and enzymatic activity to stop
d. Washes the slide

21. Which of the following represents the marked area in the histology of lymph node?

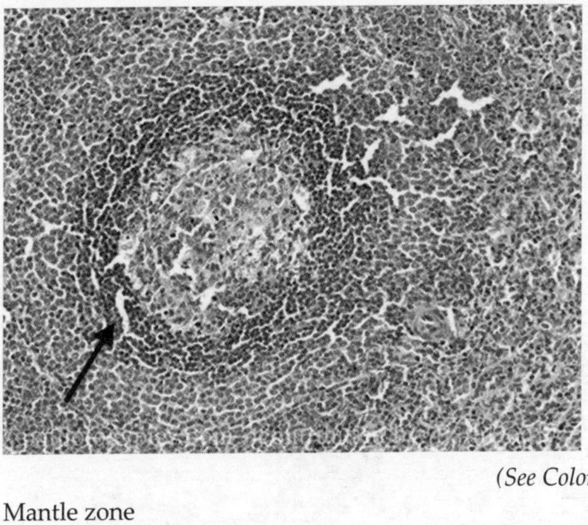

(See Color Plate 6)

a. Mantle zone
b. Marginal zone
c. Paracortical area
d. Germinal center

22. In order to avoid liver biopsy for diagnosis of fibrosis, new tests were aimed to diagnose liver fibrosis serologically. They were:

a. Serum transaminase
b. Serum laminin and serum hyaluronidase
c. Unconjugated bilirubin and GGT
d. Serum alkaline phosphatase

23. A 20-year-old boy presented with cervical lymphadenopathy. Histology of lymph node shows RS cell with vague nodule formation and background T reactive lymphocytes. The cells were positive for CD20, LCA, EMA and negative for CD15 and CD30. Diagnosis is:

a. NLPHL
b. T cell rich B cell lymphoma
c. Nodular sclerosis Hodgkin
d. CLL

24. Which of the following is accurate regarding the internal iron homeostasis in iron deficiency anemia?

a. Transferrin receptor 1—iron responding elements increases transferrin receptor mRNA concentration and synthesis
b. Ferritin mRNA concentration—iron response element increases and ferritin synthesis decreases
c. Ferritin mRNA concentration—iron response element decreases and Ferritin synthesis increases
d. Transferrin receptor 1—iron responding elements decreases transferrin receptor mRNA concentration and increases synthesis

25. A 29-year-old female with history of polyarthralgia and back ache was investigated. She had nucleolar pattern in IF. Which of the following is the best fit in her case?

a. Glomerlonephritis and heart failure
b. Raynaud phenomenon and sclerodactyly
c. Genital and oral painful ulcers
d. Joint pains with nodules on skin.

26. What is the diagnosis of the below histopathology image?

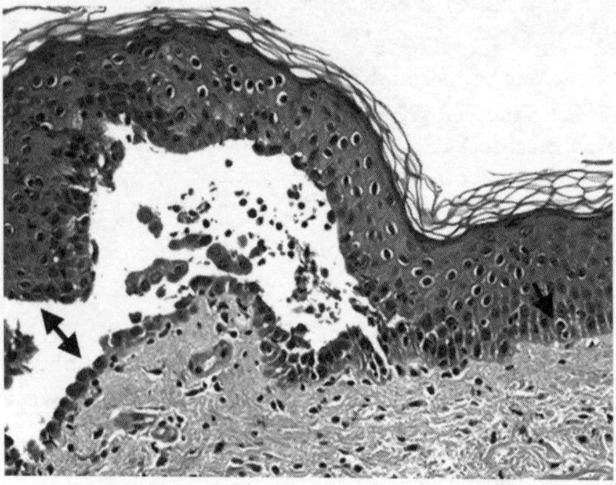

(See Color Plate 6)

a. Pemphigus
b. Leismaniasis
c. Mycosis fungoides
d. Psoriasis

27. Identify the stain done on a section of liver shown below:

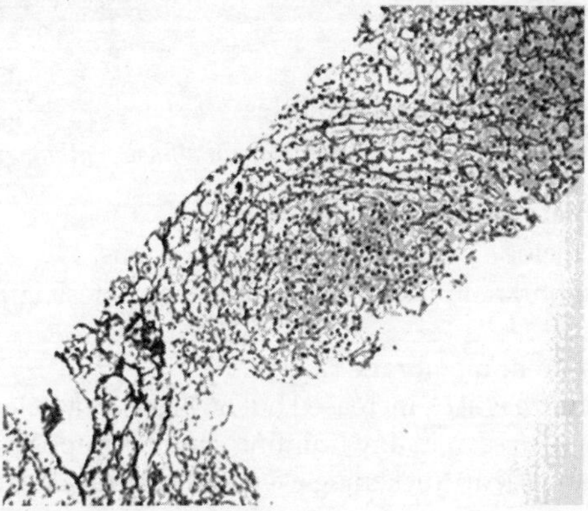

(See Color Plate 7)

a. Sweet's reticulin stain
b. Grimelins silver stain
c. Warthin starry silver stain
d. Steiner silver stain

28. An elderly male presented with history of intractable diarrhea. His bone marrow and renal biopsy as shown below. Which of the following is the most appropriate diagnosis?

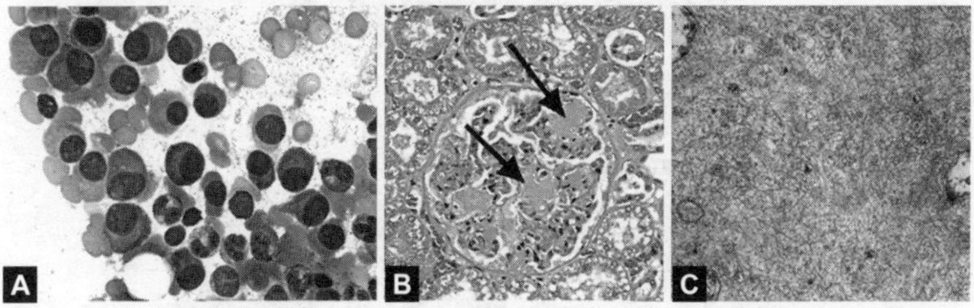

(See Color Plate 7)

a. Leishmaniasis
b. Multiple myeloma
c. Lymphoma
d. Urate nephropathy

EXPLANATIONS

1. **Ans. a. Kimmelstiel-Wilson nodules**

(Ref: Robbin's Basic Pathology 9/e p1118)

Diabetic Nephropathy:

The renal lesions include mainly—Glomerular lesions:

- Basement membrane thickening and increased mesangial matrix in ALL patients:
  - True basement membrane thickening
  - EM—The size will be increased but no black areas (electron dense deposits → as seen in any immune complex deposition)
  - EM → Can pick up thickening **even before clinical manifestation.**

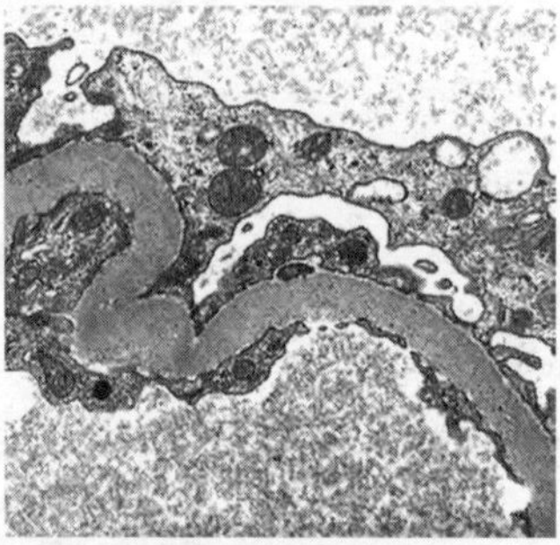

Electron micrograph of a renal glomerulus showing markedly thickened glomerular basement membrane (B) in a diabetic.

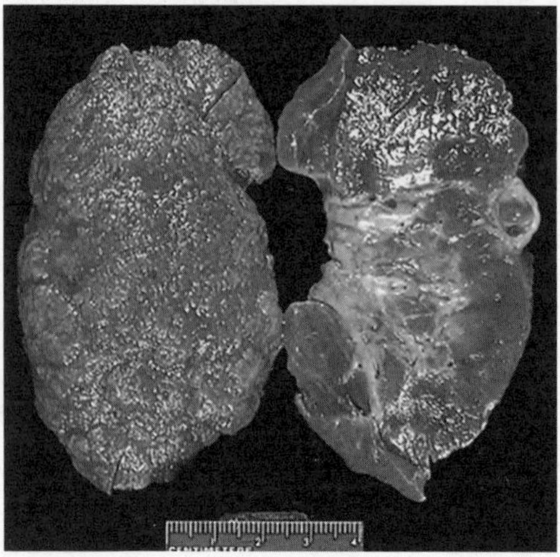

Nephrosclerosis in a patient with long-standing diabetes. The kidney has been bisected to demonstrate both diffuse granular transformation of the surface (left) and marked thinning of the cortical tissue (right).

- Diffuse glomerulosclerosis:
  - Increase in mesangial matrix associated with PAS+ basement membrane thickening, eventually obliterates mesangial cells
  - It is found in most individuals with disease of **more than 10 years duration.**
- Nodular glomerulosclerosis:
  - Intercapillary glomerulosclerosis or Kimmelstiel-Wilson disease
  - Ovoid, spherical, laminated hyaline masses in peripheral of glomerulus, PAS+, eventually obliterates glomerular tuft
  - 15% to 30% of individuals with long-term diabetes and is a major contributor to renal dysfunction.

2. **Ans. a. Antibodies against hemidesmosomes**

(Ref: Lever Dermatopathology, 10/e p273)

Antibody Targets for Pemphigus:

Diseases	Antigens	Location of Antigens
Pemphigus vulgaris		
Mucosal mainly	Desmoglein 3	Desmosomes
Mucocutaneous	Desmoglein 3	
	Desmoglien 1 (kindly note this could be a future MCQ—Desmoglien 1—mucocutaneous)	
Pemphigus foliaceus	Desmoglein1	Desmosomes

The most common bullous lesion is bullous pemphigoid—And the most common pattern of Immunofluorescence is Linera IgG deposit along basement membrane.

So, the best possible answer is (a).

3. **Ans. b. Anisocytosis**

Anisocytosis—Variation in cell size.
Poikilocytosis—Variation in cell shape.

Red cell distribution width:

- The RDW is an index of the variation in cell volume within the red cell population
- It is a parameter provided by automated hematology analyzers and is the electronic equivalent of anisocytosis or variation in red blood cell size that is judged by smear examination
- Mathematically, it is the coefficient of variation, i.e.,

RDW = (Standard deviation ÷ mean cell volume) x 100

- A high RDW indicates that the red blood cells are more variable in volume than normal
- This may be due to the presence of smaller or larger red blood cells or a combination of either scenario
- For example, increased numbers of immature red blood cells during a regenerative response to an anemia will increase the RDW, because immature anucleate red blood cells are larger than normal
- Conversely, the presence of increased numbers of smaller cells (e.g. in iron deficiency anemia) will also increase the RDW.

Normal value:

- RDW-SD 39-46 fL [1]
- RDW-CV 11.6-14.6% in adult.

Condition with increased RDW:

- Iron deficiency anemia
- Folate/vit B12 deficiency anemia.

4. Ans. a. Albumin *(Ref: Robbins Pathology, 9/e p99)*

Acute phase reactants—Inflammation, even if it is localized, is associated with cytokine-induced systemic reactions that are collectively called the acute-phase response.

Positive APPs	Negative APPs
C-reactive protein (CRP)	Albumin
Serum Amyloid A (SAA)	Transferrin
Haptoglobin (Hp)	Transthyretin
Ceruloplasmin	Retinol-binding protein
α2-Macroglobulin	
α1-Acid glycoprotein (AGP)	
Fibrinogen	
Complement (C3, C4)	

Major acute phase reactants:

- C-reactive protein (CRP), fibrinogen, and serum amyloid A (SAA) protein
- CRP and SAA, bind to microbial cell walls, and they may act as opsonins and fix complement
- Fibrinogen binds to red cells and causes them to form stacks (rouleaux) that sediment more rapidly at unit gravity than do individual red cells.

5. Ans. d. Crohn's disease *(Ref: Robbins Pathology, 9/e p798)*

The picture shows—transmural inflammation (blue part) and a overlying ulcer. The best option here is Crohn's disease.

Histopathology of Crohn's disease:

- Transmural involvement of bowel by an inflammatory process with mucosal damage
- Noncaseating, nonconfluent, sarcoid-like granulomas—occurs both involved and uninvolved segments
- Fissuring (30%) deep into muscularispropria with formation of fistulas and strictures
- Cryptitis, crypt abscess.

Crypt abscess:

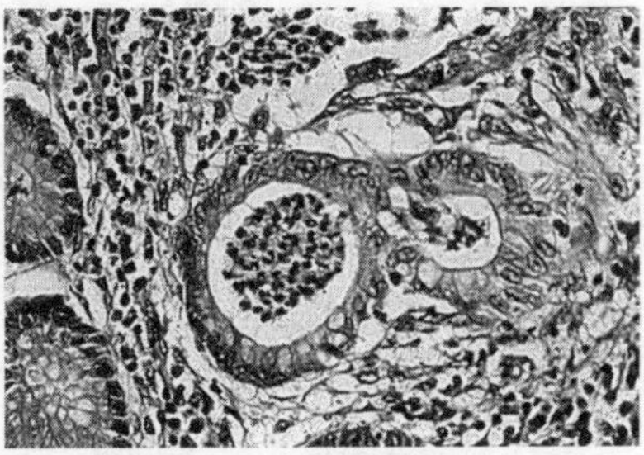

Noncaseating granuloma:

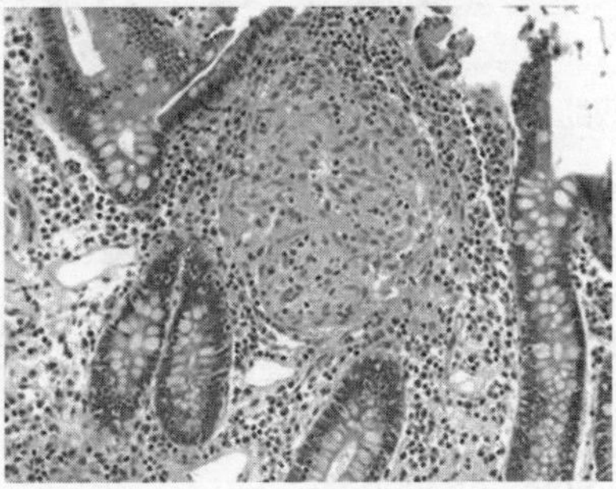

6. **Ans. c. PAX5** *(Ref: Robbins Basic Pathology 9/e p590)*

PAX5 is a B Cell marker

Below is the list of all consolidated IHC markers asked in exams.

Leukemias/Lymphomas	Enzymes positivity	CD positivity	CD negativity
AML	MPO+ Sudan black+ Chloroacetate esterase+		
AML—Monocytic	NSE+	13, 33, 34	
AML—Erythroleukemia	Glycophorin A+		

Contd...

Contd...

Leukemias/Lymphomas	Enzymes positivity	CD positivity	CD negativity
AML—M7		41, 61	
ALL	PAS+		
CLL	Surface Ig++	5, 9, 23	FMC 7
Hairy cell leukemia	TRAP+ FMC 7+	19, 20, 25, 103	5, 23
Mantle cell lymphoma	Surface Ig++	5, 19, 20	23
Follicular lymphoma	Surface Ig++	10, 19, 20, 22	5
Diffuse large B cell lymphoma		20, 45	3, 5
Anaplastic large cell lymphoma	EMA+ ALK+	3, 30	15, 20
Precursor B cell ALL	Tdt++	10, 19	
Early Pre B cell ALL	Tdt++ Cytoplasmic Ig M heavy chain	10, 19	
Burkitt's lymphoma	Surface Ig ++	10, 19, 20	
Granulocytic sarcoma	MPO+ Lysozyme++		
Hodgkin's lymphoma (Classical)		15, 30	
HL (Lymphocytic predominance type)		20, 45	30

7. Ans. d. Epigenetics *(Ref: Robbin's Basic Pathology 9/e p5)*

Epigenetics:

- Epigenetics refers to reversible, heritable changes in gene expression that occur without mutation
- They involve **posttranslational modifications** of histones and DNA methylation, both of which affect gene expression
- The major part of the genome which is not expressed are silenced by DNA methylation and histone modifications

Chromatin organization:

- Histochemically dense and transcriptionally inactive heterochromatin
- Histochemically dispersed and transcriptionally active euchromatin.

DNA methylation:

- Results in transcriptional silencing
- DNA methylation is tightly regulated by methyltransferases, demethylating enzymes, and methylated-DNA-binding proteins.

Histone modifying factors

Chromatin remodeling complexes—reposition nucleosomes on DNA, exposing (or obscuring) gene regulatory elements such as promoters:

- "Chromatin writer" complexes—denoted as marks.
- Histone marks are reversible through the activity of "chromatin erasers.
- Histone methylation and histone acetylation.

8. **Ans. b. Cell cycle will stop at G1**

(Ref: Cell cycle stops at G1, Robbins Basic Pathology 9/e p290-292)

Retinoblastoma gene:

- Ch 13q14
- Governor of cell proliferation
- **RB, a key negative regulator of the G1 /S cell cycle transition.**

Function of RB gene:

- When hypophosphorylated, RB exerts antiproliferative effects by binding and inhibiting E2F transcription factors that regulate genes required for cells to pass through the G1-S phase cell cycle checkpoint
- Normal growth factor signaling leads to RB hyperphosphorylation and inactivation, thus promoting cell cycle progression
- **So a problem in phosphorylation will result in RB gene result in a active RB → stopping the cell cycle at G1S transition.**

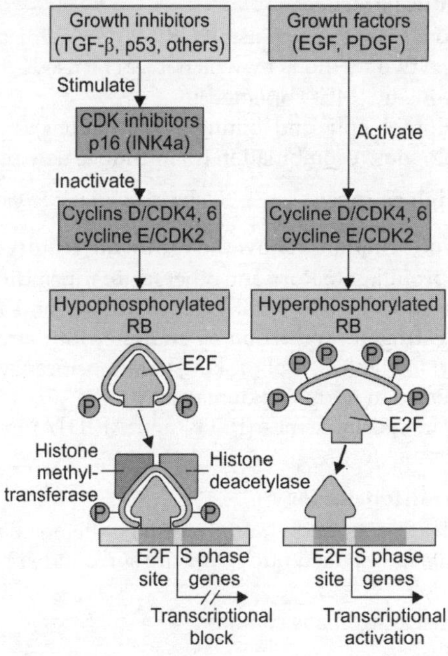

Knudson **"two-hit" hypothesis of oncogenesis:**

- Two mutations (hits), involving both alleles of RB are required to produce retinoblastoma
- In familial cases, children inherit one defective copy of RB gene in the germline (the first hit), and the other copy is normal. The other hit happens sporadically to produce the tumor.

9. **Ans. b. CRISPR** *(Ref: Robbins Basic Pathology, 10/e p5-6)*

CRISPR:

- ***CRISPR***-Cas9 is a genome editing tool
- CRISPR Cas9 system is essential in adaptive immunity in select bacteria enabling the organisms to respond to and eliminate invading genetic material (asked in JIPMER may 2017)
- There are three types of CRISPR mechanisms identified. Of which type II is the most commonly explored
- CRISPRs are transcribed and processed into an RNA sequence that binds and directs the nuclease Cas9 to a sequences (e.g., a phage), leading to its cleavage and the destruction of the phage
- Gene editing repurposes this process by using artificial guide RNAs (gRNAs) that bind Cas9 and are complementary to a DNA sequence of interest. Once directed to the target sequence by the gRNA, Cas9 induces double-strand DNA breaks.

CRISPR in medical practice

Though it's a long way to go in using CRISPR for medical practice. The following are the two methods by which it can be used.

- Repair is done by (MCQ oriented):
  - Non-Homologous end joining (for mutations)
  - Homologous recombination (to introduce new sequence).

10. **Ans. a. High estrogen** *(Ref: Robbin Basic Pathology 10/e p721)*

The endometriotic implants show the following features:

- Release of proinflammatory and other factors, including PGE2, IL-1β, TNFα, IL-6 and -8, NGF, VEGF, MCP-1, MMPs, and TIMPs
- **Increased estrogen production by endometriotic stromal cells**, due in large part to high levels of the key steroidogenicenzyme aromatase, which is absent in normal endometrial stroma
- Mutations in specific genes (PTEN and ARID1A) in endometriotic cysts—Potential future question.

Endometriosis Histopathology:

- Endometrial glands, endometrial stroma or hemorrhage
- Stromal cells have naked nuclei and are surrounded by reticulin and spiral arterioles
- Smooth muscle stroma is common

Chocolate cyst

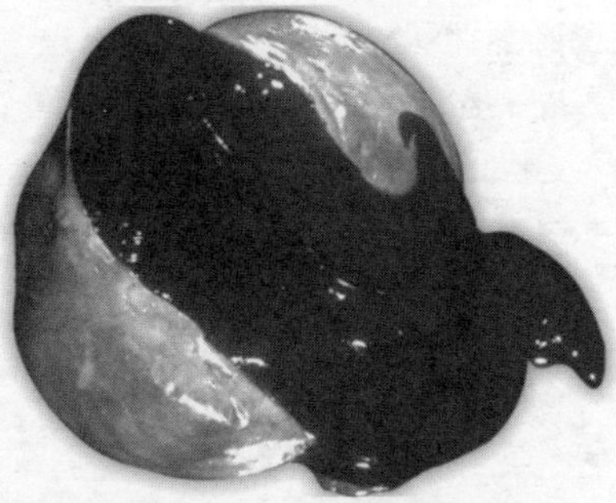

Glands and stroma

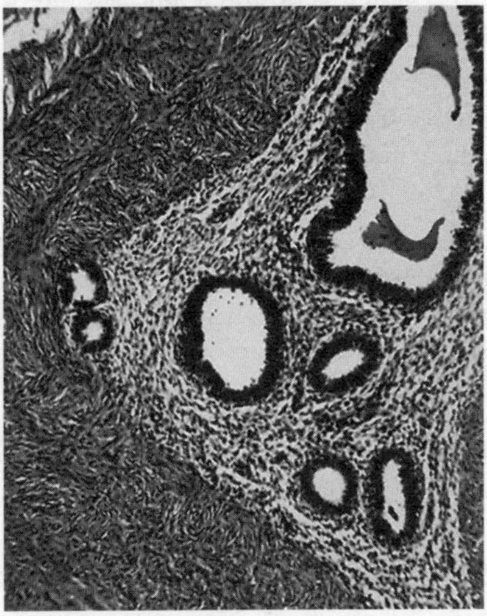

11. Ans. b. Inflammatory myofibroblastic tumor

(Ref: Robbins Basic Pathology, Chapter Neoplasia)

ALK gene:

- Anaplastic lymphoma kinase (ALK) – Location: 2p23
- It's also seen in:
  - Adenocarcinoma lung.
- Neuroblastoma
- Inflammatory myofibroblastic tumor
- Diffuse large B cell lymphoma
- It's negative in fibromatosis, one of the important thing to differentiate from difficult cases of inflammatory myofibroblastic tumor.

Targeted therapy against ALK—Crizotinib

Image-based question: (A. H and E × DLBCL, B. IHC × ALK)

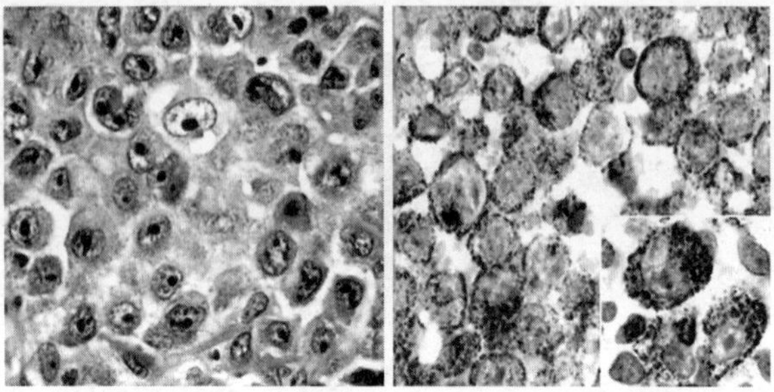

12. Ans. b. AIRE *(Ref: Robbins Basic Pathology, p145)*

The above process is called central tolerance, where the self-reacting T cells are presented to the thymus to prevent autoimmunity.

Central tolerance

Immature self-reactive T and B lymphocyte clones that recognize self antigens during their maturation the central (or generative) lymphoid organs (the thymus for T cells and the bone marrow for B cells) are killed or rendered harmless.

T cells and central tolerance:

- When immature lymphocytes encounter the antigens in the thymus, many of the cells die by apoptosis. This process,called negative selection or deletion
- A protein called autoimmune regulator (AIRE) stimulates expression of some "peripheral tissue-restricted" self antigens in the thymus and is thus critical for deletion of immature T cells specific for the seantigens
- Mutations in the AIRE gene are the cause of an autoimmune polyendocrinopathy.

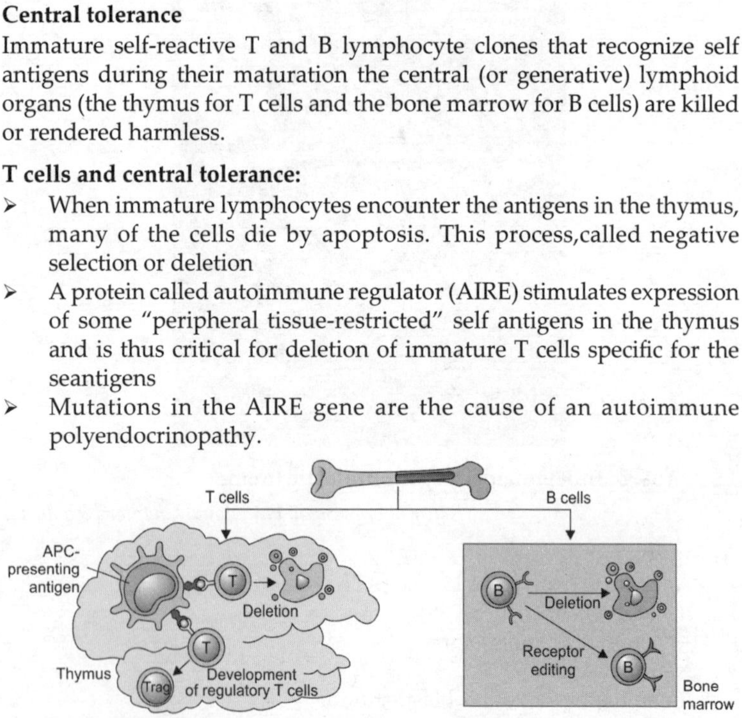

13. Ans. b. B cells, Dendritic cells, NK cells

(Ref: Robbins Basic Pathology, 9/e p191)

"Any cell with MHC type II will be called a professional antigen presenting cell"

Professional APC's	Amateur APC's
Expresses MHC II	Do not express MHC II, activated by cytokines
Good amount of costimulatory molecules	Less number of costimulatory molecules
Dendritic cells Macrophages B cells M cells—seen in intestine NK cell	Fibroblasts Thymic epithelial cells Glial cells Endothelial cells

14. Ans. a. SOX11 *(Ref: Robbins Pathology 9/e p592)*

Mantle cell lymphoma:

- Tumor cells resemble the normal mantle zone B-cells
- Have the translocation t(11; 14).
- Intestinal involvement—**lymphomatous polyposis**

Lymphomatous polyposis:

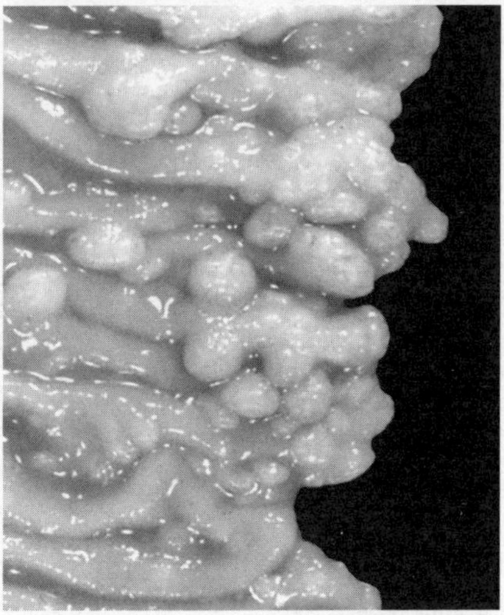

Microscopy:

- Three patterns of tumor infiltration: (1) diffuse replacement of entire lymph node, (2) infiltration into expanded mantle zone or (3) vague nodular pattern
- Tumor cells are monotonous small lymphocytes resembling centrocytes/mantle cells with scant cytoplasm, cleaved, slightly irregular or round nuclei; condensed chromatin
- Tumor cells have no nucleoli; no large cells, no proliferation centers

IHC:

- Positive stains—CD5, CD19 (strong), CD20 (strong), cyclin D1/BCL1 (variable nuclear staining since cells are at different stages of cell cycle) also CD22, CD43, CD79a, FMC7, surface IgM or IgD, kappa or lambda, BCL2
- SOX 11 positive in cyclin D1 negative mantle
- Negative stains—CD23, usually CD10; also BCL6, CD11c, TdT, T cell antigens.

15. Ans. b. Membranous glomerulopathy

(Ref: Robbins Pathology, 9/e p915, 920)

Rule out options:

- Minimal change disease—it is does not have and Immunofluorescence(IF) finding
- FSGS—Its more of a light microscopic finding and not IF or electron microscopic based diagnosis.

Disease	Light microscopy	Fluorescence	Electron microscopy	Presentation
Post streptococcal GN	Proliferation of endothelail and mesangial cells	IgG, IgM, C3 deposits in mesangium		Nephritic syndrome
RPGN – I	Crescents in glomeruli	Linear GBM deposits of IgG and C3		Severe glomerular injury with worst diagnosis
RPGN – II	Crescents in glomeruli	Lumpy bumpy granular pattern of staining		
RPGN – III	Crescents in glomeruli	No Ig or Complement deposits in GBM		
Membranous glomerulopathy	Diffuse capillary wall thickening	Granular IgG, C3	Subepithelial deposits	Nephrotic syn
Minimal change disease	Lipid deposit in tubules	Negative	Loss of foot process of podocytes	MCC of nephrotic syn in children
Focal segmental glomerulosclerosis	Focal and segmental sclerosis and hyalinosis	Focal—IgM and C3	Loss of foot process of podocytes, Epithelial denudation.	MCC of nephrotic syn in adults and AIDS pts

Contd...

Contd...

Disease	Light microscopy	Fluores-cence	Electron microscopy	Presenta-tion
Membrano-proliferative glomerulone-phritis Synonymous with mesan-giocapillary glomerulone-phritis. Type 1 MPGN Type 1 MPGN –	Mesangial pro-liferation, BM thickening and splitting – tram track Deposition of immune complexes IgG and complement Dense deposit disease	IgG + C3 and C1q + C4 C3, no C1q or C4	Subendothe-lial deposits	
Ig A nephropa-thy (Burger's disease)	Mesangial widening and proliferation	Mesangial deposition of IgA, C3 and properdin		Recurrent hematuria/ proteinuria
Alport syn-drome	Presence of foam cells in interstitial cells		Irregular foci of thickening and thinning in GBM with splitting and lamination of lamina densa	Basket Weave appearance in EM
Good pasture syndrome	Focal necrosis, intra-alveolar hemor-rhage, type II pneumocyte hypertrophy		Linear depos-its of Ig along alveolar septa and GBM	Anti—BM antibody

Subepithelial	Acute glomerulonephritis Membranous GN Heymann GN RPGN (some cases)
Subendothelial	MPGN type 1 SLE Acute GN (early stages)
Basement membrane	MPGN type 2
Mesangial	IgA nephropathy HSP

Now, the EM shows a subepithelial deposits with IF showing dense granular deposits the diagnosis is Membranous Glomerulonephritis.

16. Ans. a. ALL *(Ref: Robbins Pathology, 9/e p611)*

- The picture is that of a lymphoblast. Lymphoblasts will be 3-4x larger than a mature RBC, high nuclear to cytoplasmic ratio, round nucleus with immature chromatin (not clumped), prominent nucleoli, cytoplasm is scant, light blue and lacks granules.

FAB classification of ALL

L1 ALL	L2 ALL	L3 ALL
Best prognosis	Worst prognosis	Very worst prognosis
Small homogeneous blast Scanty cytoplasm Indistinct nucleoli	Large heterogeneous blast Abundant cytoplasm Intended nuclei	Large homogeneous blast Abundant cytoplasm Cytoplasmic vacuolation

Immunological classification of ALL

Features	B cell lineage (more common)	T cell lineage (Less common)
Immunophenotyping	Immunoglobulins, CD19 and CD20	CD1, CD2, CD5, CD7, CD3, CD4, CD8
Associated disease pattern	Pancytopenia	Mediastinal mass, lymphadenopathy, splenomegaly
Genetics	Loss of function mutation in PAX 5, E2A and EBF or balanced t(12;21) affecting Tel and AML 1 genes	Gain of function mutation in NOTCH 1 gene

Prognostic factors in ALL

Good prognosis	Bad prognosis
Age 2-10 years Female sex L1 cell Peripheral blast count <1,00,000 Pre B cell phenotype Absence of mediastinal mass Hyperdiploidy or t(12;21) Trisomy 4, 7 and 10	Age <1 or >10 years Male sex L2 or L3 cell Peripheral blast count >1,00,000 Pre T cell phenotype Presence of mediastinal mass Pseudodiploidy or t(9;22) or t(8;14) or t(4;11)

17. Ans. c. EBV positive—DLBL

(Ref: Hematological Malignancies, WHO, p223)

EBV positive DLBL	EBV positive mucocutaneous ulcer (WHO 2016 entity
Immunocompetent	Immunocompromised
Patients > 50 years old	30-50 years old
70% of patients present with extranodal disease (most commonly skin, lung, Tonsil (our case) and stomach) with or without simultaneous lymph node	Circumscribed ulcer involving oro-pharyngeal mucosa, skin, or gastro-intestinal tract (not mass forming)
The cells are positive for CD20, CD79a, IRF4/MUM1 positive, EBV LMP1 and EBNA negative, CD15 negative. Back-ground are predominantly T lympho-cytes	B-cell immunophenotype with uniform expression of CD30, MUM1, PAX5, and OCT-2, and variable CD20, CD45, CD15, CD79a, and BCL-6 expression

Analysing the question now – Clearly, it's immune competent patient with a tonsilar mass forming ulcer with IHC profile like that of EBV positive DLBL, with large cells in the picture.

18. Ans. a. Barrett esophagus

(Ref: Robbins Pathology, 9/e p757)

- Barrett's esophagus is the metaplastic change in the esophageal lining in which the normal squamous epithelium is changed to columnar epithelium due to prolonged gastroesophageal reflux (GERD)
- Columnar metaplasia, glandular metaplasia, goblet cell metaplasia
- Definite diagnosis is made only when columnar mucosa contains **the intestinal goblet cells, which will be positive for PAS, Alcian blue (mucin stain).**

Types of Barrett esophagus

- **Long-segment:** Barrett's mucosa extends 3 cm or more
- **Short-segment:** Barrett's mucosa extends less than 3 cm
- **Ultra short-segment:** Barrett's mucosa extends less than 1 cm.

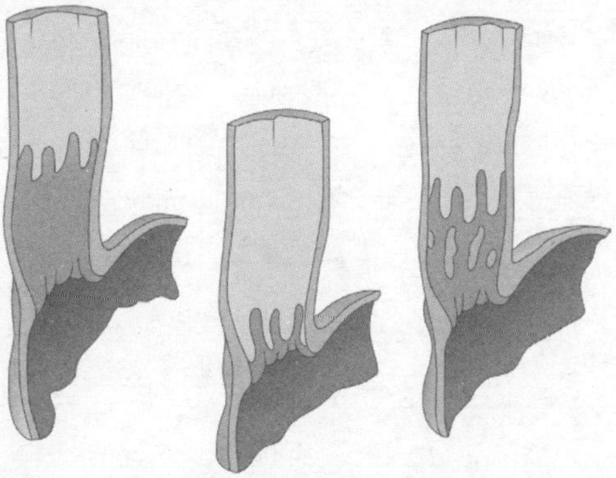

19. Ans. c. 3 *(Ref: Harrison 19/e p396)*

Reticulocyte count has two corrections:

- Correction for the degree of anemia (absolute reticulocyte count)
- Correction for the prolonged duration of stay of reticulocyte in peripheral smear
- The value you get at the end of two corrections is called reticulocyte production index (RPI), based on which anemia's are classified into hypoproliferative or hyperproliferative

So let's have a look at this question

Data:

- Hemoglobin – 5%
- Reticulocyte – 9%

Absolute reticulocyte count → Reticulocyte count × Hb of patient/Standard HB

- = 9 × 5/15
  = 9/3 = 3

Absolute reticulocyte count = 3%

20. Ans. c. Causes metabolic and enzymatic activity to stop

(Ref: Bancroft's Histochemical Techniques, p90-98)

Acetone free methanol is the fixative in leishman stain:

- Romanowsky stains are neutral stains composed of a mixture of oxidized methylene blue (azure) dyes and Eosin Y
- The azures are basic dyes that bind acid nuclei and result in a blue to purple color
- The acid dye, eosin, is attracted to the alkaline cytoplasm, producing red coloration.

Routine fixatives in histopathology

Most commonly used	10% Neutral buffered formalin
Electron microscopy	Glutaraldehyde
Trephine biopsy – Bone marrow	Zenker's fluid (AZF fixative)
Brain	Formalin ammonium chloride
Adrenal biopsy	Orth's fluid
PAP smear	Ethanol
Connective tissue	10% NBF; Zenker's; Helly's Bouin's
DNA/RNA	Ethanol

Glycogen	Carnoy's or Gendre's
Glycoproteins	Alcoholic formalin Carnoy's
Mitochondria	Carson-Millonig's
Uric acid crystals	Absolute ethanol

21. Ans. a. Mantle zone *(Ref: Robbins Pathology, 9/e p583)*

This is a very basic question in histology of lymph nodes. Let's see the normal histology of lymph nodes.

- Normal lymph node
- Cortex → Lymphoid follicles and paracortical areas
- Medulla → Predominantly blood vessels.

Structures in a follicle

- **Germinal center**: round/oval zone containing pale staining cells, surrounded by darker cells
- **Mantle zone**: small unchallenged B cells surrounding pale staining germinal centers
- **Marginal zone**: light zone surrounding follicles; contains postfollicular memory B cells derived after stimulation of recirculating cells from T cell dependent antigen; named "marginal cells" due to location.

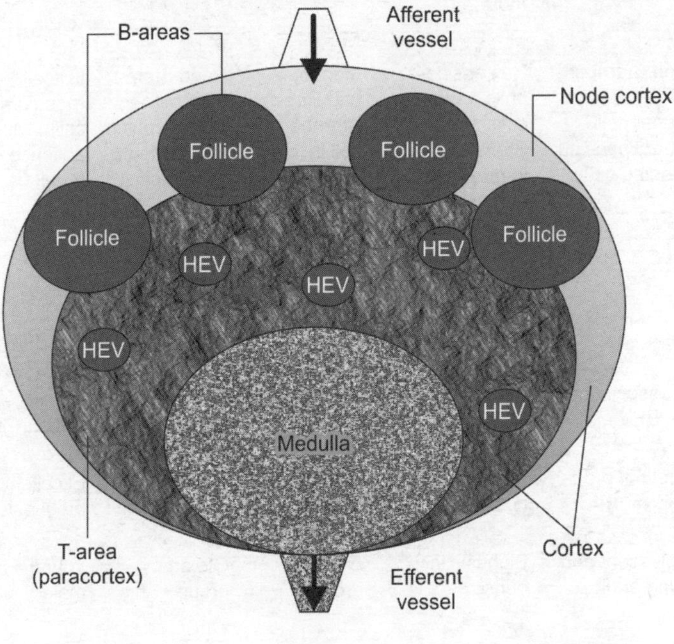

IHC:

- Germinal centers have strong dense BCL6 and CD10 expression
- Terminal deoxynucleotidyl transferase (TdT) is expressed by premature B and T cells
- B cells express CD19, CD20, CD79a
- Antigen stimulated B cells with the capacity to differentiate toward plasma cells express MUM1/IRF4 and CD138
- T cells express CD2, CD3, variable CD4 and CD8.

22. Ans. a. Serum laminin and serum hyaluronidase

(Ref: Journal of Hepatology)

- ELF Score: Enhanced Liver Fibrosis score (ELF) (Siemens Healthcare, Erlangen, germany) patented formula combining age, hyaluronate, MMp-3 and TIMP-1

23. Ans. a. NLPHL *(Ref: Robbins Pathology, 9/e p606)*

This is classical description of NLPHL. (Nodular lymphocyte predominant Hodgkin lymphoma).

Nodular sclerosis	Mixed cellularity	Lymphocyte rich	Lymphocyte depleted	Lymphocyte predominant
Most common type of HL	Most common type of HL in India		Associated with HIV	
M = F	M > F	M > F	M > F	M > F
Reed Sternberg cell variant in lacunar cell (Clear space surrounding cell)	Has eosinophils & plasma cells and Reed Sternberg cell in maximum numbers	Mononuclear and Reed Sternberg cell in low numbers	Reed Sternberg cell—pleomorphic, mummified & necrobiotic	LH cells (pop corn cells) with absence of B cell
Cells are CD 15^+ and CD 30^+	Cells are CD 15^+ and CD 30^+	Cells are CD 15^+ CD 30^+ and CD 20^-	Cells are CD 15^+ and CD 30^+	Cells are CD 15^+, CD 30^+, CD 20^+, BCL6$^+$ and EMA$^+$
No association with EBV	Associated with EBV	Associated with EBV	Associated with EBV	No association with EBV
Excellent prognosis	Very good prognosis	Good to excellent prognosis	Poor prognosis	Excellent prognosis
Adolescent and young adult	Biphasic incidence	Old age group	Old age group	Young males

24. Ans. a. Transferrin receptor 1—iron responding elements increases transferrin receptor mRNA concentration and synthesis

Investigations for Iron Deficiency Anemia:

Test	Interpretation
MCV	MCV <80 fL
MCH	Low <27.5 picograms/red cell
MCHC	Low < 295 g/L (<29.5 g/dL)
Red cell distribution width (RDW)	RDW >14.6%
Peripheral blood smear	Microcytic, hypochromic red cells
Reticulocyte count	Low
Serum iron	Decreased
Total iron-binding capacity (TIBC)	Increased
Transferrin saturation	Transferrin saturation less than 16%
Serum ferritin	Low (a serum ferritin <12 nanograms/mL is diagnostic of iron deficiency)
Urinalysis	Blood may be present if cause of blood loss is from the renal tract

	Decreasing iron	Increasing iron
Iron uptake	↑	↓
Transferrin receptor synthesis	↑	↓
Transferrin receptor mRNA concentration	↑	↓
Iron storage	↓	↑
Feritin synthesis	↓	↑
Ferritin mRNA concentration	No change	No change

25. Ans. b. Raynaud phenomenon and sclerodactyly

(Ref: Robbins Basic Pathology, 9/e p226)

Patterns in Antinuclear Antibody (ANA) testing

Diffuse or homogenous	dsDNA, histone	SLE, DLE
Rim/peripheral	Ds DNA	SLE
Speckled	Sm	SLE
	SS-A, SS-B	Sjogren syndrome
Nucleolar	Nucleolar RNA	Scleroderma

Systemic sclerosis is characterized by:

- Chronic inflammation thought to be the result of autoimmunity
- Widespread damage to small blood vessels
- Progressive interstitial and perivascular fibrosis in the skinand multiple organs.

Scleroderma is classified into two broad categories:

- Diffuse scleroderma, characterized by widespread skin involvement at onset, with rapid progression and early visceral involvement
- Limited scleroderma, in which the skin involvement is often confined to fingers, forearms, and face.

Crest syndrome:

- Limited disease can develop a combination of calcinosis, Raynaud phenomenon, esophageal dysmotility, sclerodactyly, and telangiectasia (abbreviated as CREST syndrome, more specifically will have centromere pattern of staining)

Nucleolar Staining

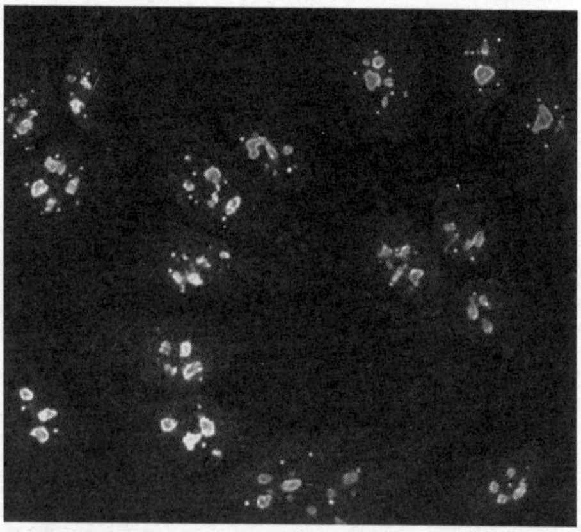

Centromere Staining

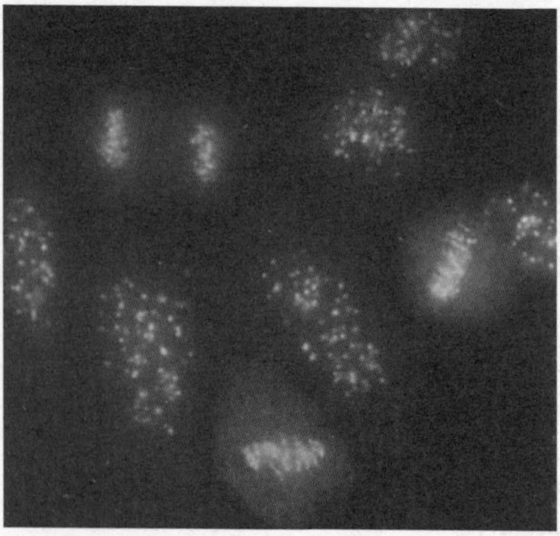

26. Ans. a. Pemphigus *(Ref: Robbins Pathology 9/e p1167)*

Pemphigus Vulgaris:
- Suprabasal blister formation
- Row of tombstone appearance.

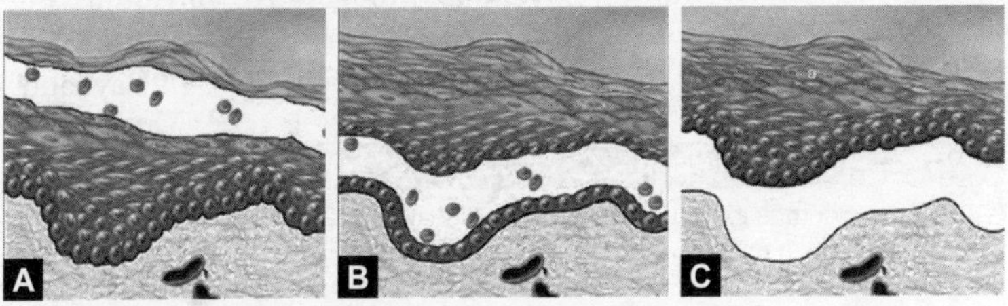

Features of Pemphigus Vulgaris:
- Large painful, nonitchy flaccid bulla
- Mucocutaneous lesion
- Nikolsky sign—Positive
- Morbidity/Mortality – 2° infections
- Rare association with intestinal cancer, Castleman's disease, Thymoma, Myasthenia gravis, SLE.

27. Ans. a. Sweets reticulin stain

(Ref: Bancroft Histochemical Techniques, p180)

Reticulin stain
- Demonstrates reticular fibers and basement membrane material
- Not related to reticulum cells
- Reticular fibers: thin, usually type III collagen, widespread in connective tissue throughout the body.

Staining procedure:

There are two procedures by which reticulin stain is done
- Gordon and Sweet's reticulin stain (most commonly done)
- Gomori reticulin stain.

Below is the picture of myelofibrosis in marrow:

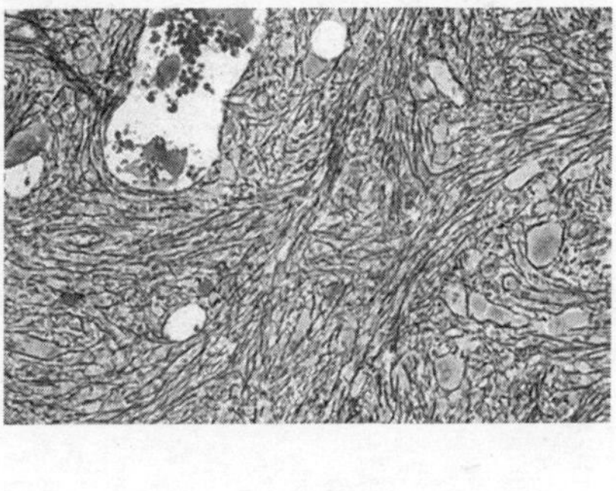

28. Ans. b. Multiple myeloma *(Ref: Robbins Pathology, 9/e p595)*

- First picture → Increase in plasma cells in marrow
- Second picture → Kidney biopsy with pink deposits in glomerulus
- Third picture → Fibrils in electron microscope
- Diagnosis → **Multiple myeloma, probably AL amyloidosis of kidney.**

Criteria for multiple myeloma—Old criteria—still questions come on this basis.

Major criteria	Minor criteria
❍ Plasmacytomas in tissue biopsy ❍ Marrow plasmacytosis with > 30% plasma cells ❍ M spikes in serum electrophoresis ❍ > 3.5 g/dl for IgG and > 2 g/dl for IgA or 1 g/dl of κ or λ light chain excretion on urine electrophoresis in absence of amyloidosis	❍ Lytic bone lesions ❍ Marrow plasmacytosis 10-30% ❍ Monoclonal globulin spikes present in lower level

Myeloma Defining events/Biomarkers of Malignancy: New criteria

Clonal bone marrow plasma cells ≥ 10% or plasmacytoma plus one of these:	
	2-y Incidence of Organ Damage, %
Clonal marrow plasma cells ≥ 60%	95
Ratio of involved to uninvolved serum free light chain ≥ 100	80[a]
≥ 2 focal bone lesions ≥ 5 mm on MRI	70–80

Biomarkers of malignancy (MDEs):

- 60% or greater clonal plasma cells on bone marrow examination
- Serum involved/uninvolved free light chain ratio of 100 or greater, provided the absolute level of the involved light chain is at least 100 mg/L (a patient's "involved" free light chain—either kappa or lambda—is the one that is above the normal reference range; the "uninvolved" free light chain is the one that is typically in, or below, the normal range)
- More than one focal lesion on MRI that is at least 5 mm or greater in size.

PHARMACOLOGY

QUESTIONS

1. **Which of the following is an antidote for fibrinolytic therapy?**
   a. Streptokinase
   b. Epsilon aminocaproic acid
   c. Protamine
   d. Heparin
2. **Which of the following disease modifying anti-rheumatoid drugs increases extracellular adenosine?**
   a. Hydroxychloroquine
   b. Methotrexate
   c. Leflunomide
   d. Sulfasalazine
3. **All are idiosyncratic reactions of carbamazepine *except*:**
   a. Stevens-Johnson syndrome
   b. Rash
   c. Blurred vision
   d. Agranulocytosis
4. **Lente insulin is:**
   a. 30% amorphous 70% crystalline
   b. 70% amorphous 30% crystalline
   c. Other name of NPH insulin
   d. Only 70% amorphous
5. **A 12-year-old boy came with complaints of 4 hypopigmented patches on back and on left arm. The patches had loss of sensation. Which of the following is the treatment for this case?**
   a. Rifampicin (450 mg) + Dapsone (50 mg) + Clofazimine (150 mg) monthly and 50 mg daily
   b. Rifampicin (600 mg) + Dapsone (150 mg) only
   c. Rifampicin (450 mg) + Dapsone (50 mg) + Clofazimine (150 mg) monthly and 50 mg alternate days
   d. Rifampicin (600 mg) + Dapsone (150 mg) + Clofazimine (300 mg) monthly and 50 mg daily
6. **A 40-year-old person who was diabetic with CKD stage 5 on insulin wanted to change to oral drugs. Which of the following can be given to the patient safely in renal failure without change in dose?**

a. Linagliptin
b. Sitagliptin
c. Vildagliptin
d. Saxagliptin

7. **Oseltamivir (Tamiflu) acts by which of the following mechanisms?**
a. Inhibition of RNA dependent DNA polymerase
b. Acts by inhibiting viral M2 receptors
c. Acts by inhibiting neuraminidase
d. Acts by causing apoptosis of cells

8. **A drug was given IV at a rate of 1.6 mg/min. The clearance of the drug is 640 mL/min. The half life of the drug is 1.8 hour. Calculate the plasma concentration of the drug:**
a. 0.002 mg/mL
b. 3.55 mg/mL
c. 2.88 mg/mL
d. 0.004 mg/mL

9. **Which of the following is a P-glycoprotein substrate?**
a. Ketoconazole
b. Itraconazole
c. Azithromycin
d. Rifampicin

10. **Which of the following is the mechanism of action of protease inhibitor in HIV?**
a. Inhibits proviral RNA synthesis
b. Inhibits assembly of viral proteins
c. Inhibits conversion of RNA to DNA
d. Blockage in entry of the virus into the cell

11. **Drug of choice for prophylaxis of pneumocystis jirovecii in an immunocompromised patient is:**
a. Cotrimoxazole
b. Amoxicillin
c. Dexamethasone
d. Cephalosporin

12. **A known case of epileptic patient on *Levetiracetam*. He is now seizure free for 2 years. But he developed agitation and anger issues interfering with his day to day activities as a result of the drug intake. Which of the following is the best case scenario here?**
a. Stop levetiracetam and start on a different antiepileptic
b. Discontinue the drug as he is seizure free
c. Slowly taper the drug over next 6 months
d. Continue levetiracetam since a 5-year seizure free interval is needed

13. A 27-year-old female came with complaints of greenish discharge-vagina and on examination she had strawberry vagina. Which of the following is the treatment for her?

a. Metronidazole
b. Doxycycline
c. Fluconazole
d. Amoxicillin

14. Which of the following is most bactericidal antileprotic drug?

a. Ofloxacin
b. Amoxicillin
c. Erythromycin
d. Ciprofloxacin

15. In an animal model how will you show vasomotor reversal of Dale?

a. Stimulation of alpha1 followed by stimulation of beta2
b. Block of alpha1 followed by stimulation of beta2
c. Stimulation of alpha1 followed by block of beta2
d. Stimulation of beta1 receptor followed by block of beta2 receptor

16. If a patient is given 200 mg drug, 75 mg excreted in 90 min and if the drug follows first order kinetics. How much drug will remain after 6 hours?

a. 6.25 mg
b. 12.5 mg
c. 25 mg
d. 50 mg

17. Storage of drugs in tissue is suggested by:

a. Small volume of distribution
b. Large volume of distribution
c. Excretion in urine
d. Excretion in saliva

EXPLANATIONS

1. **Ans. b. Epsilon aminocaproic acid**

(Ref: Goodman and Gilman, p865-868)

What is Fibrinolysis?

- Fibrinolysis is the breakdown of a fibrin clot.
- Plasmin is the enzyme that breaks down fibrin. It is activated from inactive plasminogen by tissue plasminogen activator (tPA) and urokinase.
- Tissue plasminogen activator (tPA) and urokinase are inhibited by plasminogen activator inhibitor-1 and plasminogen activator inhibitor-2 (PAI-1 and PAI-2).

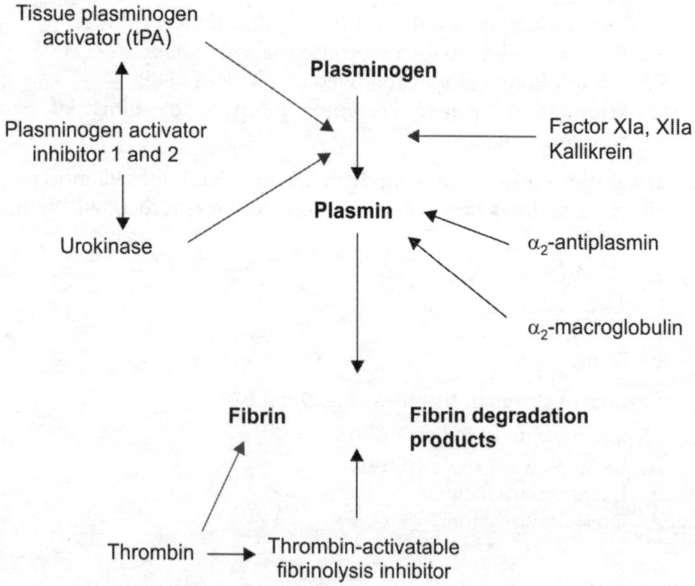

There are two antidotes for fibrinolysis: EACA and Tranexamic acid.

- Epsilon-aminocaproic acid (EACA):
  It is an analogue of the amino acid lysine: combines with the lysine binding sites of plasminogen and plasmin so that the latter is not able to bind to fibrin and lyse it. It is a specific antidote for fibrinolytic agents.
- **Tranexamic acid** binds to the lysine binding site on plasminogen and prevents its combination with fibrin and is 7 times more potent.

2. Ans. b. Methotrexate *(Ref: Goodman and Gilman, p960)*

Methotrexate and Extracellular adenosine.

- MTX inhibitsAICAR transformylase, which in turn decrease degradation of AICAR and the levels increase.
- Increase in AICAR -> inhibits Adenosine deaminase (ADA) -> Increases extracellular Adenosine.
- This increase in the adenosine also plays a role in the anti-inflammatory property of Methotrexate.
- **Precaution**: All patients should take **folic acid 1 mg daily or folinic acid 5 mg weekly** to reduce the risk of certain side effects, such as upset stomach, sore mouth, low blood cell counts, and abnormal liver function.

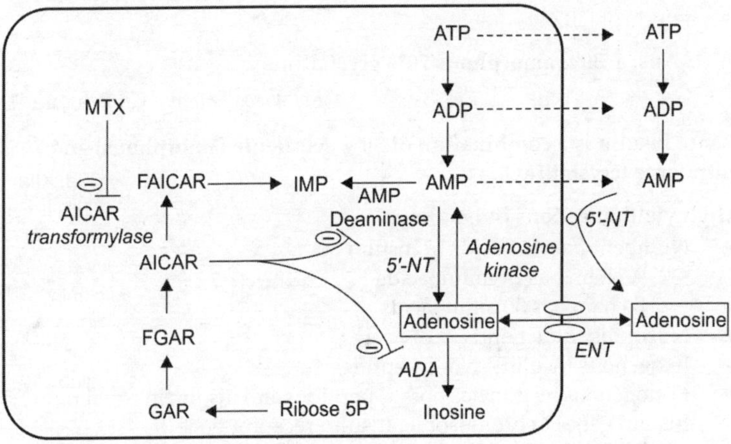

DMARD:

- DMARDs work to suppress the body's overactive immune and/or inflammatory systems.
- They take effect over weeks or months and are not designed to provide immediate relief of symptoms.
- Most common DMARD used: The most common DMARDs are **methotrexate, sulfasalazine, hydroxychloroquine, and leflunomide.** Less frequently used medications include gold salts, azathioprine, and cyclosporine.

3. Ans. c. Blurred vision *(Ref: Goodman and Gilman, p585)*

Carbamazepine:

- Carbamazepine inhibits sustained repetitive firing by blocking use-dependent sodium channels.

- Pain relief is believed to be associated with blockade of synaptic transmission in the trigeminal nucleus and seizure control with reduction of post-tetanic potentiation of synaptic transmission in the spinal cord.
- Carbamazepine also possesses anticholinergic, central antidiuretic, antiarrhythmic, muscle relaxant, antidepressant (possibly through blockade of norepinephrine release), sedative, and neuromuscular-blocking properties.

Idiosyncratic reactions of Carbamazepine:

- People with **HLA-B*1502 allele** have increased propensity for idiosyncratic reactions like SJS and TEN and the drug should be avoided.
- Blurred vision, diplopia, ataxia and vertigo are dose related adverse effects of CBZ.

4. **Ans. a. 30% amorphous 70% crystalline**

(Ref: Goodman and Gilman, p1241)

Lente insulin is a combination of 30% semilente (amorphous) and 70% ultralente (crystalline).

High yield questions in insulin:

- Number of amino acids in insulin 51
  - A chain has 21 aminoacids
  - B chain has 30 aminoacids
- No. of disulfide bonds—3
- Exogenous insulin—No C peptides
- Endogenous insulin has both C peptides and insulin in equal ratio 1:1
- Insulin gene11 chromosome, Insulin receptor gene19

Classification of insulin:

Rapid acting	Short acting	Intermediate acting	Long acting
Insulin lispro Insulin aspart Insulin glulisine	Regular (soluble) insulin	Insulin zinc suspension or Lente Neutral protamine hagedorn (NPH) or isophane insulin	Protamine zinc insulin (PZI) Insulin glargine

5. **Ans. c. Rifampicin (450 mg) + Dapsone (50 mg) + Clofazimine (150 mg) monthly and 50 mg alternate days**

(Ref: Govt guidelines. Gov. in)

The diagnosis is Multibacillary and age 12. Look at the guidelines below:

Type of leprosy	Drugs used	Frequency of administration adults (children in bracket)	Dosage (adult) 15 years & above	Dosage (Children 10–14 years)#	Dosage children Below 10 years*	Criteria for RFT
MB leprosy	Rifampicin	Once monthly	600 mg	450 mg	300 mg	Completion of 12 monthly pulses in 18 Consecutive months
	Clofazimine	Monthly	300 mg	150 mg	100 mg	
	Dapsone	Daily Once	100 mg	50 mg	25 mg	
	Clofazimine	Daily for adults (every other day for children)	50 mg	50 mg (alternate day, not daily)	50 mg (weekly twice)	
PB leprosy	Rifampicin	Once monthly	600 mg	450 mg	300 mg	Completion of 6 montly pulses 9 consecutive months
	Dapsone	Daily	100 mg	50 mg	25 mg daily or 50 mg alternate day	

*For children below 10 years, doses (as per kg body wt) should be provided losse (capsules/tablets) after opening appropriate BCP.

6. Ans. a. Linagliptin

(Ref: Katzung, Basic & Clinical Pharmacology, p1090)

Gliptins Pharmacokinetics

- Linagliptin lowers HbA1c by 0.4–0.6% when added to metformin, sulfonylurea, or pioglitazone. The dosage is 5 mg daily and since it is primarily excreted via the bile, no dosage adjustment is needed in renal failure.
- Saxagliptin is given orally as 2.5–5 mg daily. The drug reaches maximal concentrations within 2 hours (4 hours for its active metabolite). It is minimally protein bound and undergoes hepatic metabolism by CYP3A4/5. The major metabolite is active, and excretion is by both renal and hepatic pathways. The terminal plasma half-life is 2.5 hours for saxagliptin and 3.1 hours for its active metabolite. Dosage adjustment is recommended for individuals with renal impairment.

Side effects of OHA (oral hypoglycemic agents)

Group	Main side effect
Alpha-glucosidase inhibitor	Flatulence/Dyspepsia
SGLT–2 inhibitors	UTI & vaginal infections
Gliptins	Stevens-Johnson syndrome
Thiazolidinediones	Water retention/Macular edema

Contd...

Contd...

Group	Main side effect
Insulin	Hypoglycemia/Lipodystrophy
Chlorpropamide	SIADH/Disulfiram like reaction
Tolbutamide	Hepatotoxicity
Metformin	Vit. B12 deficiency
Phenformin	Lactic acidosis
Meglitinides	Hypoglycemia

7. Ans. c. Acts by inhibiting neuraminidase

(Ref: Goodman and Gilman, p1609)

Oseltamivir

- Oseltamivir acts by **inhibiting viral neuraminidase** enzyme which is responsible for release of mature virions.
- It is given by oral route.
- Zanamivir—Inhalational

Infection	Drug	Route	Dosage
Influenza A and B: Treatment	Oseltamivir	Oral	Adults: 75 mg bid x 5 d Children 1–12 years: 30–75 mg bid, depending on weight, x 5 d
	Zanamivir	**Inhaled orally**	Adults and children ≥7 years: 10 mg bid x 5 d
	Amantadine	Oral	Adults: 100 mg qd or bid x 5–7 d Children 1–9 years: 5 mg/kg per day (maximum, 150 mg/d) x 5–7 d
	Rimantadine	Oral	100 mg qd or bid x 5–7 d in adults

High yield questions in influenza:

- Influenza A—Hemagglutinin and neuraminidase is strain specific
- Influenza—Major epidemics are due to antigenic SHIFT, Antigenic drift is gradual antigenic
- Change over a period of time. Antigenic shift is due to genetic recombination of virus
- H1N1 swine flu was found on—2009
- Influenza is associated with—Myositis and Rhabdomyolysis
- Most serious complication of Influenza B—Reye syndrome
- Amantadine and rimantadine are active against—Influenza A only
- Segmented RNA virus—Influenza virus
- M protein in orthomyxovirus maturation—Serves as a recognition site for nucleocapsid at the inner face of plasma membrane.

8. **Ans. a. 0.002 mg/mL**

(Ref: K.D. Tripathi, Essentials of Medical Pharmacology, p8)

Maintenance dose:

- It is calculated by the below formula.

Maintenance dose (D) = Plasma Concentration (C_p) * Clearance (Cl)

- C_p = D/Cl
  C_p = [1.6 mg/min] / [640 mL/min]
  C_p = 0.0025 mg/mL

9. **Ans. a. Ketoconazole**

(Ref: KD. Tripathi, Essentials of Medical Pharmacology, p15)

- **P-glycoprotein 1**/multidrug resistance protein 1 (MDR1)
- It is an **ATP-dependent efflux pump** with broad substrate specificity.
- Plays an important role in drug metabolism.

Medications that act as substrates, inhibitors or inducers of P-gp		
Substrate	**Inhibitors**	**Inducers**
❍ Cyclosporine ❍ Dipyridamole ❍ Digoxin ❍ Diltiazem ❍ Losartan ❍ Quinidine ❍ Tacrolimus	❍ Amiloride ❍ Amiodarone ❍ Atorvastatin ❍ Carvedilol ❍ Cyclosporine ❍ Digoxin ❍ Diltiazem ❍ Dipyridamole ❍ Doxazosin ❍ Felodipine ❍ Lidocaine ❍ Lovastatin ❍ Nifedipine ❍ Propafenone ❍ Propranolol ❍ Quinidine ❍ Simvastatin ❍ Spiroanolactone ❍ Verapamil	❍ Aspirin ❍ Cyclosporine ❍ Paclitaxel ❍ Reserpine

10. **Ans. b. Inhibits assembly of viral proteins**

(Ref: Goodman and Gilman, p1645)

Protease inhibitor – Anti retroviral

Protease inhibitors (PIs) block protease (an HIV enzyme). By blocking protease, PIs prevent new (immature) HIV from becoming a mature virus that can infect other CD4 cells.

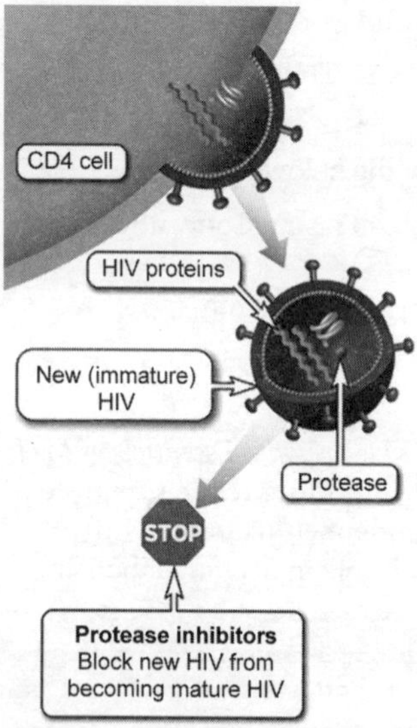

- HIV protease inhibitors are peptide-like chemicals that competitively inhibit the action of the **virus aspartyl protease**.
- Indinavir (IDV), Nelfinavir (NFV), Saquinavir (SQV), Ritonavir (RTV) and Lopinavir are the drugs used.
- All are extensively metabolized by CYP3A4.

11. Ans. a. Cotrimoxazole *(Ref: Goodman and Gilman, p1434)*

Pneumocystis jiroveci pneumonia:

- History of dyspnea on exertion or nonproductive cough of recent onset (within the past 3 months).
- Chest film evidence of diffuse bilateral interstitial infiltrates or gallium scan evidence of diffuse bilateral pulmonary disease.

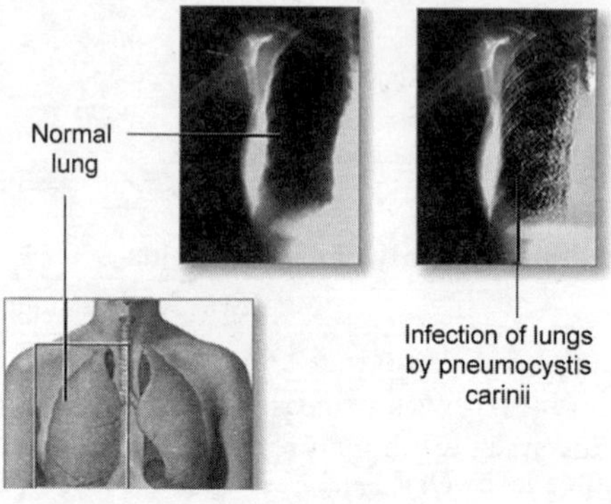

Cup and saucer appearance – GMS stain

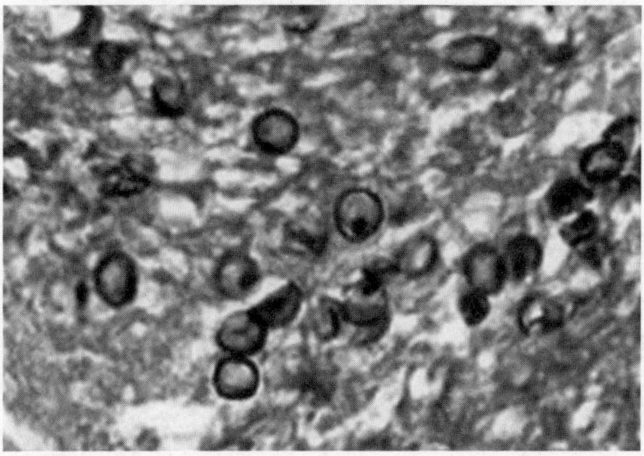

Treatment:

- High-dose therapy (trimethoprim 15–20 mg/kg/d plus sulfamethoxazole 75–100 mg/kg/d in three or four divided doses) is effective for this severe infection in patients with AIDS.
- Prophylaxis with 800 mg sulfamethoxazole and 160 mg trimethoprim once daily or three times a week is effective in preventing pneumonia caused by this organism in patients with AIDS.

12. Ans. c. Slowly taper the drug over next 6 months

(Ref: Goodman and Gilman, p600)

- Levetiracetam can cause mood disturbances and patient may complain of dizziness, agitation, and insomnia.
- Abrupt stoppage of Levetiracetam can lead to rebound seizures.

Levetiracetam:

Mechanism of action: binds to a protein on the presynaptic neuronal plasma membrane and stops release of excitatory NT, e.g. glutamate

Used in

- Partial seizures with or without secondary generalization
- Adjunctive therapy of:
  - Partial seizures with or without secondary generalization
  - Primary generalized tonic-clonic seizures in idiopathic generalized epilepsy
  - Myoclonic seizures in juvenile myoclonic epilepsy in patients > 12 years

Precautions:

- Learning disability, history of psychiatric problems—increase risk of behavioral problem.

- Treatment with drugs that lower the seizure threshold —use combinations cautiously, if at all.
- Renal—Reduce dose in renal impairment.
- Pregnancy: Plasma concentrations may decrease during pregnancy and may increase rapidly postpartum.
- Breastfeeding—Excreted in breast milk.

Adverse effects

- **Common**- behavioral effects, e.g. depression, aggression, anxiety, drowsiness, dizziness, ataxia-diplopia, insomnia.
- Rare: SJS, TEN , multi-organ hypersensitivity syndrome
- Thrombocytopenia

13. Ans. a. Metronidazole

(Ref: K.D. Tripathi, Essentials of Medical Pharmacology, p 837)

This patient is suffering from Trichomonas Vaginalis

Rx:

Trichomonas vaginalis infection

- Metronidazole is DOC for trichomoniasis. 2 g single dose is preferred or 400 mg BD/TDS can be given for 7 days.

Treatment options for Sexually Transmitted Disease:

Disease	1st choice of drugs
Gonorrhea	
No-penicillinase producing	Amoxicillin 3 g oral or Ampicillin 3.5 g oral + Probenecid 1g oral dose
Penicillinase producing	Ceftriaxone 250 mg i.m. or Cefuroxime 250 mg i.m or Azithromycin 1.0 g oral
Granuloma inguinale	Tetracycline 500 mg QID oral × 3 weeks or Doxycycline 100 mg BD oral × 3 weeks or Azithromycin 500 mg OD oral × 7 days
Chancroid	Ceftriaxone 0.25 g i.m. single dose or Azithromycin 1.0 g oral single dose or Erythromycin 0.5 g QID oral × 7 days
Chlamydia trachomatis	
Nonspecific urethritis	Azithromycin 1 g oral single dose or Doxycycline 100 mg BD oral × 7 days
Lymphogranuloma	Azithromycin 1.0 g oral weekly × 3 weeks or Doxycycline 100 mg BD oral × 3 weeks

14. Ans. a. Ofloxacin *(Ref: Goodman and Gilman, p1566)*

Ofloxacin, a fluoroquinolone is given to leprosy patients as intermittent ROM (Rifampicin +Ofloxacin + Minocycline) regimen.

- Of all the above drugs only ofloxacin is given to treat leprosy as it has been found to hasten bacteriological and clinical response.

Classification of antileprotic drugs:

- Sulfone: Dapsone (DDS)
- Phenazine derivative: Clofazimine
- Antitubercular drugs: Rifampin, Ethionamide
- Other antibiotics: Ofloxacin, Minocycline, Clarithromycin.

Ofloxacin

- Ofloxacin as a component of MDT and found it to hasten the bacteriological and clinical response.
- 99.9% bacilli were found to be killed by 22 daily doses of ofloxacin monotherapy.
- Dose: 400 mg/day.

15. Ans. b. Block of alpha1 followed by stimulation of beta2

(Ref: Principles of Physiology, D. Prmanik, p173)

Vasomotor reversal of Dale is a phenomenon is exaggerated fall in BP after alpha receptor blockade. Phenomenon is based on the biphasic action of adrenaline on BP. Adrenaline acts on alpha1 receptors at low dose and beta2 at high dose. When its given at a dose of say 5 mg IV, it will stimulate alpha1 receptors first leading to increase in BP, then when its dose gets reduced by metabolism beta2 receptors get stimulated which leads to fall in BP. Now when alpha blockers like phentolamine is given this will block all alpha receptors thereby preventing the initial action of adrenaline. Therefor all the available adrenaline are bound to act on beta2 receptors, thereby leading to exaggerated fall in BP.

Concept 1:

- Alpha1 receptor stimulation: Vasoconstriction
- Alpha2 receptor stimulation: Vasodilatation
- Beta1 receptor stimulation: Increase cardiac force of contraction → Can increase BP
- Beta2 receptor stimulation: Vasodilatation

Concept 2:

- Beta receptors are more sensitive to adrenaline than alpha receptors → Even low dose of adrenaline can stimulate beta receptors

16. Ans. c. 25 mg

- First order kinetics means t1/2 is constant.
- This means time taken for reduction of 50% of concentration remains throughout the drug's life time in plasma.

- Time take for 75 mg elimination is 90 minutes.
- Thus the time taken for 200 mg → 100 mg = 2 hours.
- Therefore in 6 hours (3 t1/2), 25 mg of drug will be remaining in plasma 200 → 100 → 50 → 25 (three t1/2 → 3×2 hours = 6 hours)

17. Ans. b. Large volume of distribution

(Ref: Goodman and Gilman, p32)

Concept:
- Drugs with small VD → Confined to vascular compartment
- Drugs with large VD → Extravascular compartments like adipose tissue, muscle, bone, etc.

Volume of distribution:
- Volume V into which drug gets immediately and uniformly distributed

$$V = \frac{\text{Dose administered i.v.}}{\text{Plasma concentration}}$$

Factors governing volume of distribution:
- Lipid: water partition coefficient of the drug
- pK_a value of the drug
- Degree of plasma protein binding
- Affinity for different tissues
- Fat: Lean body mass ratio, which can vary with age, sex, obesity, etc.
- Diseases like CHF, uremia, cirrhosis.

MICROBIOLOGY

QUESTIONS

1. Which of the following parasite's life cycle is shown below?

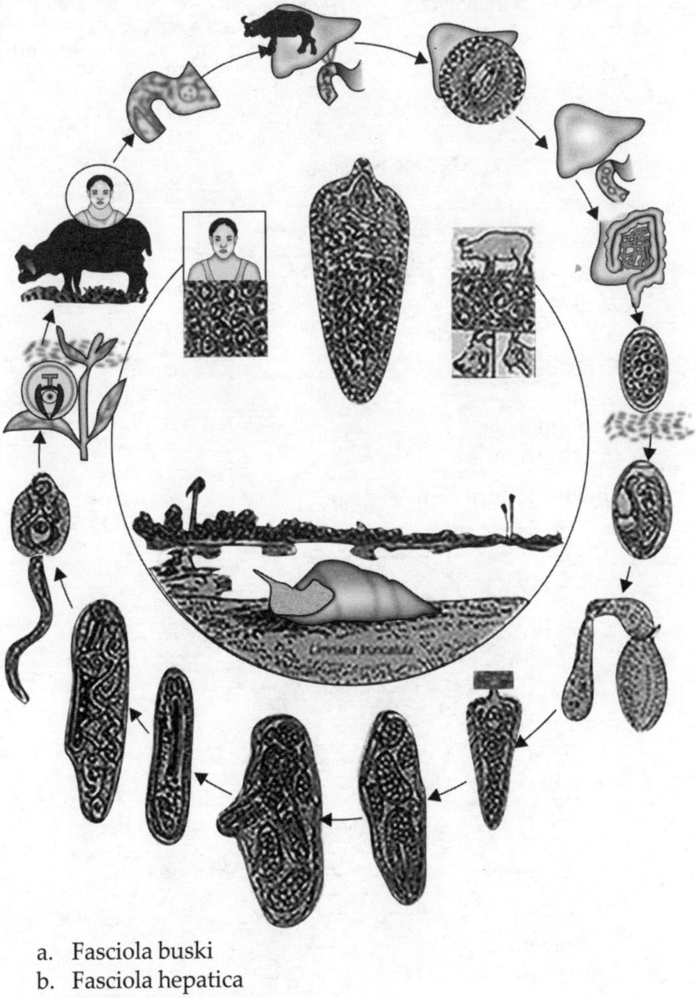

a. Fasciola buski
b. Fasciola hepatica
c. Clonorchis sinensus
d. Pargaonimus westermani

2. **Which of the following fits to the life cycle image given below?**

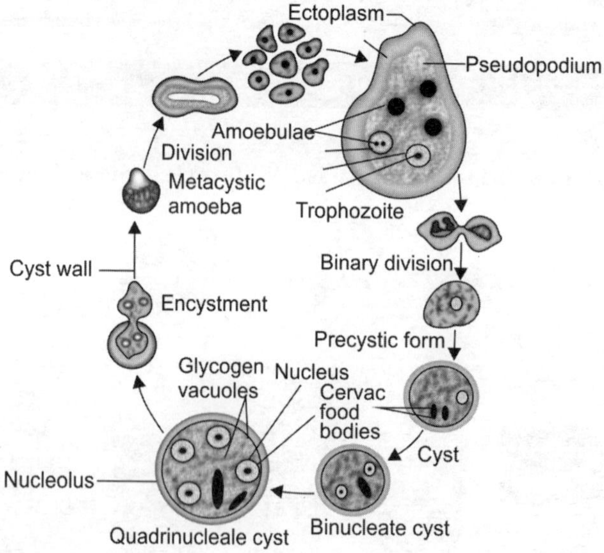

a. E. histolytica
b. B. coli
c. A. duodenale
d. E. vermicularis

3. **The below picture shows egg of:**

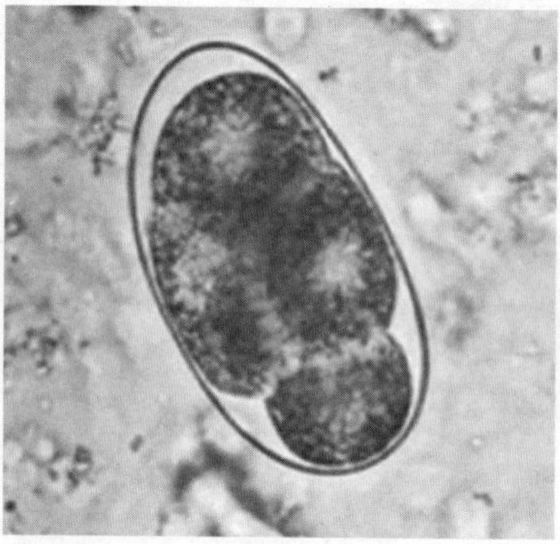

(See Color Plate 7)

a. A. duodenale
b. E. vermicularis
c. A. lumbricoides
d. Strongyloides stercoralis

4. **The following is a picture from scrapping of genital ulcer. Your diagnosis is:**

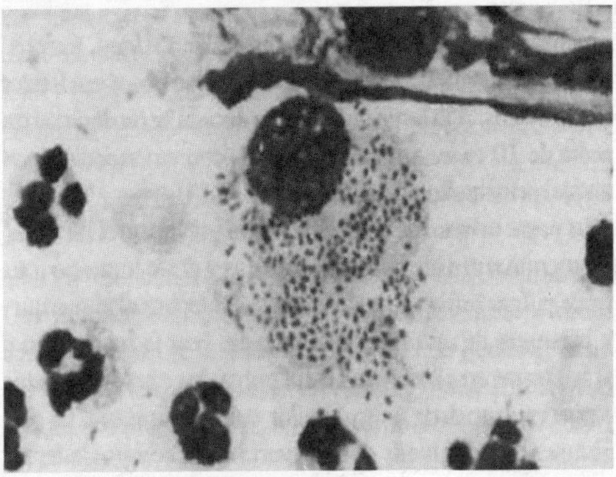

(See Color Plate 8)

a. Klebsiella granulomatis
b. Hemophilus ducreyi
c. Neisseria gonorrhoea
d. Chlamydia trachomatis

5. **Papain cleaves the immunoglobulin molecule into:**

a. 1 Fc and 2 Fab fragments
b. 2 FC and 1 FAB fragments
c. 1 Variable chain and 1 constant chain
d. I FAB and one hypervariable region

6. **Identify the below organism:**

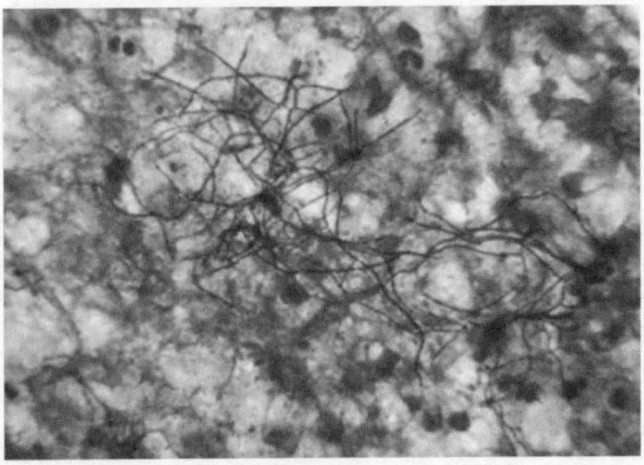

(See Color Plate 8)

a. Nocardia sp.
b. Mycobacterium tuberculosis
c. Mycobacterium leprae
d. Actinomyces sp.

7. **Which of the following staphylococcal infection is not toxin mediated?**
   a. Toxic shock syndrome
   b. Staphylococcal scalded skin syndrome
   c. Food poisoning
   d. Septicemia

8. **A 20-year-old male with history of fever and enlarged lymph nodes and sore throat was suspected to have infectious mononucleosis and was ordered a Paul Bunnel test. Which of the following is the principle of the test?**
   a. Heterophile antibody test
   b. Neutralization reaction
   c. Complement mediated cell damage
   d. Agglutination reaction

9. **Rhinosporidium seeberi belongs to:**
   a. Fungus
   b. Bacteria
   c. Aquatic protistan protozoa
   d. Virus

EXPLANATIONS

1. **Ans. b. Fasciola hepatica** *(Ref: TB of parasitology – Chaterjee – p187-190)*

The above is the exact picture in the exam. Taken directly from text book. The life cycle is that of fasciola hepatica.

Approach to this kind of question is easy if you know the life cycle theory.

- Look at the organ affected
- Look at the animal involved (here it's snail, this is enough to narrow down the options)
- Look at the infective form (can help in narrowing options)
- Look at the egg – (single, quadri or multiple)

Fasciola hepatica - Sheep liver fluke comes under Trematodes/flukes

- Adult worms reside in the biliary passages of the liver of sheep, goat, cattle and man
- Eggs are large, elliptical, operculate, light yellowish brown colored. Each egg has an immature larva, the miracidium which extends to the shell margins without a clear space
- Ova cannot be distinguished from Fasciolopsis buski – (important for future mcq's)
- Infective form: Metacercariae encysted on water plants that are ingested by humans
- Definitive host: Sheep, goat, cattle and man
- First intermediate host: Snails
- Lab diagnosis: Detection of eggs in stool or in bile obtained by duodenal intubation

Fasciola Buski:

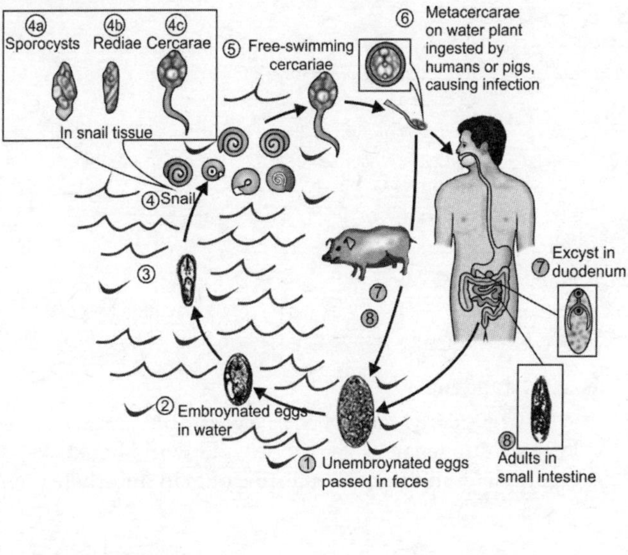

Eggs of Fasciola: Unemryonated eggs:

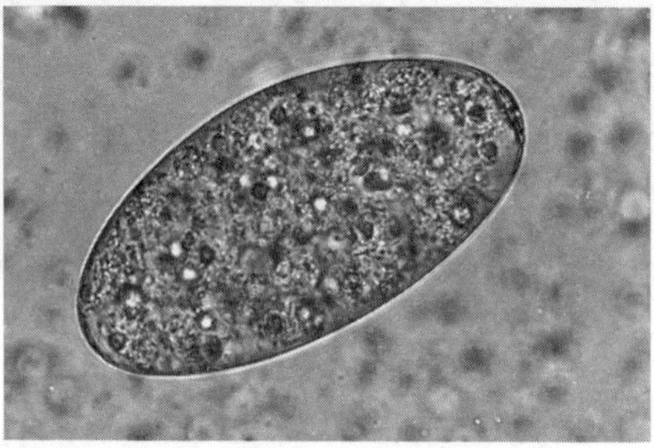

2. **Ans. a. E. histolytica**

(Ref: Medical Microbiology. Patrick Murray, 8/e p69)

Entamoeba histolytica – Three morphological forms available – Trophozoite, Pre cyst, Cyst

- Habitat: Trophozoites reside in mucosa and submucosa of large intestine of man
- Trophozoite: The invasive form present in tissues; it has red blood cells, leucocytes and tissue debris in the food vacuoles of endoplasm; motility is active, purposeful and unidirectional with the help of pseudopodium
- Infective form: Mature quadrinucleate cysts
- Pathogenicity: Intestinal amoebiasis and extra intestinal amoebiasis (Liver abscess M/c) and its complications due to rupture

Features	E. histolytica	E. coli
Trophozoite		
Motility	Active	Sluggish
Pseudopodia	Finger shaped, rapidly extruded	Short, blunt, slowly extruded
Inclusions	RBC, no bacteria	Bacteria and no RBC
Nucleus	Not clearly visible, eccentric	Visible in unstained films
Nuclear membrane	Delicate	Thick
Cysts		
Size in microns	10-15	10-30
Nucliei	4, central karyosome	8, eccentric karyosome
Chromatidial bars	1-4, with rounded ends	Splinter like with angular ends

3. **Ans. a. A. duodenale**

(Ref: Medical Microbiology by Patrick Murray, 8/e p858)

- Ancylostoma duodenale – Nematode – old world hookworm
- Adult worm lives in the small intestine of man (mostly Jejunum)

- Eggs: Eggs are oval or elliptical in shape; colorless – non bile stained; surrounded by a thin transparent hyaline shell; has a segmented ovum with four blastomeres; Eggs are similar for both hookworms – Ancylostoma duodenale and Necator americanus

Difference between ankylostoma and necator:

- A. duodenale live on average 1–3 years and N. americanus live 3–10 years
- A. duodenale can infect by ingestion of eggs as well as via the skin, whereas N. americanus infects only through the skin
- Migrating larvae of N. americanus grow and develop in the lungs, whereas those of A. duodenale do not
- A. duodenale possesses the ability to remain within the host as a larval stage for many months before finally developing to an adult, thus bridging seasons which are inappropriate for transmission.

Egg of enterobius vermicularis:

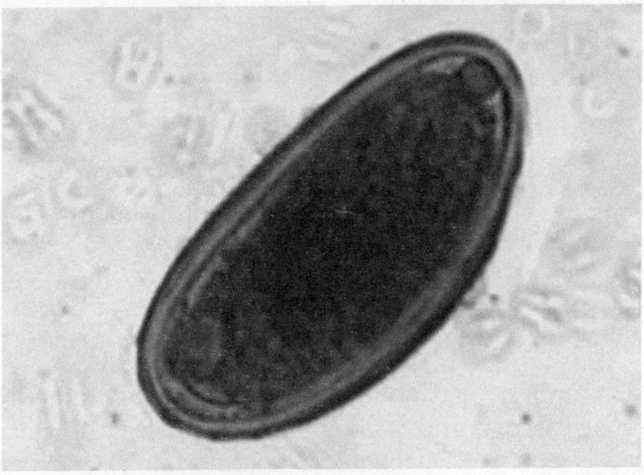

Eggs of ascaris (fertilized and unfertilized):

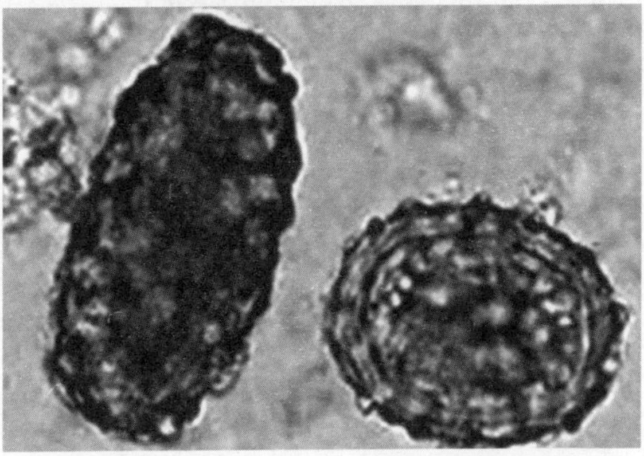

Strongoloides egg:

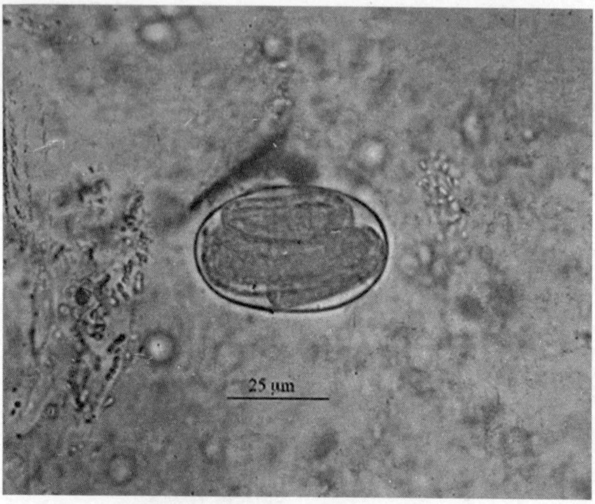

4. **Ans. A. Klebsiella granulomatis**

(Ref: Jawetz Medical Microbiology – 27/e p794)

The three major genital ulcer diseases are syphilis, genital herpes, and chancroid

- H.ducreyi – Chancroid – School of fish appearance – not seen here
- N.gonorrhea – and chlamydia trachpmatis
- Available option – Best one is Klebsiella granulomatis

Klebsiella granulomatis (Calymmatobacterium granulomatis)

- The causative organism of granuloma inguinale is difficult to culture
- Diagnosis requires visualization of dark-staining Donovan bodies on tissue crush prep (shown as in the above picture)
- With clinical information of genital ulcer and gram negative rods inside macrophage suggest diagnosis of Klebsiella granulomatis

Hemophilus – School of fish appearance

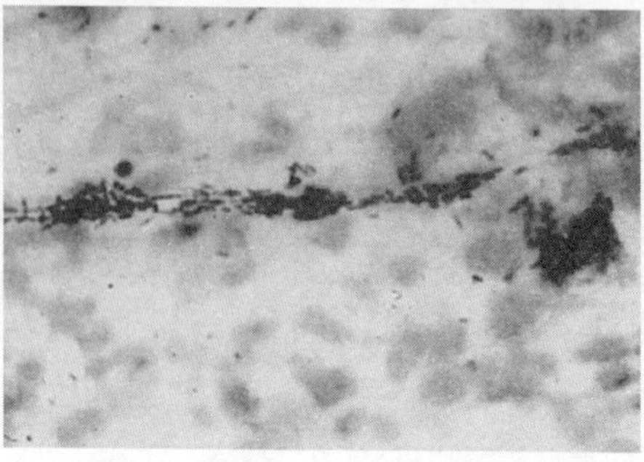

Gonorrhea in neutrophils

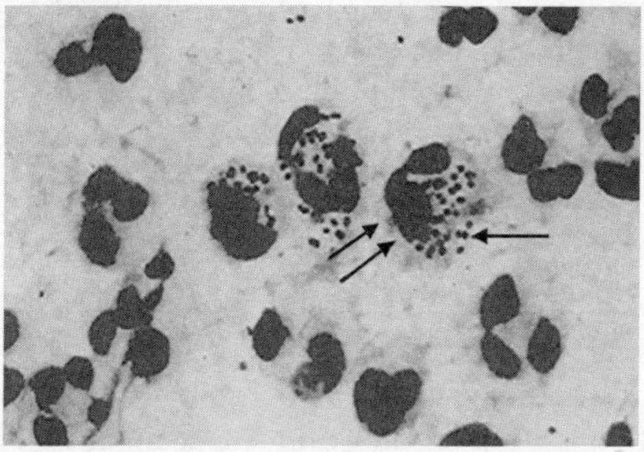

5. Ans. a. 1 Fc and 2 Fab fragments

(Ref: Jawetz medical microbiology. 25/e p129)

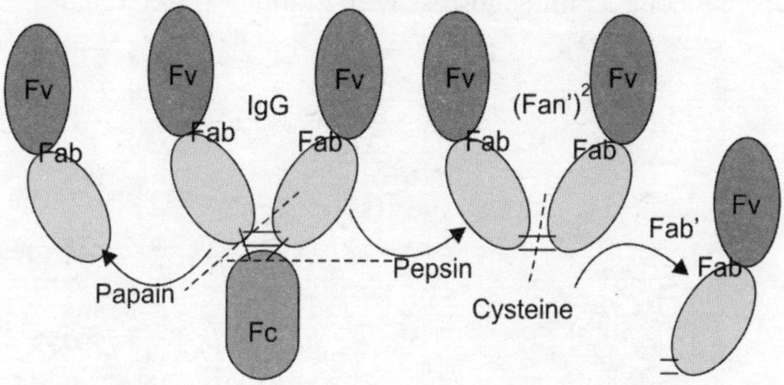

Papain digestion

- Enzyme papain cleaves the hinge region on the N- terminal side of the inter-heavy chain disulfides and this result in the formation of three fragments. (Two fragments containing the variable region and one fragment containing the CH2 and CH3 regions).
- The two fragments containing the variable region are called; Fab fragments, (i.e. fragment antigen binding) as they have the antigen-binding sites.
- The third fragment comprises the carboxyl-terminal portions of both heavy chains held together by disulfides.

Pepsin digestion:

- Enzyme pepsin cleaves the immunoglobulin on the carboxy-terminal side of hinge region resulting in one large fragment called F (ab') 2. The F (ab') 2 has two Fab fragments linked by disulfide bonds.
- The Fc region is extensively degraded by pepsin, and usually no intact Fc fragment remains after pepsin digestion.

6. **Ans. a. Nocardia sp.** *(Ref: Jawetz medical microbiology. 25/e p182)*

- The above acid fast stain (blue background with pink bacilli) shows Nocardia asteroides–Gram positive branching filaments – causes nocardiasis–in immunocompromised individuals

Nocardia:

- Gram+, aerobic, non-spore forming, non- motile, branching filamentous rod.
- Partially acid fast
- Immunocompromised pts, cancer pts.

Diseases:

- Cavitary bronchopulmonary Nocardiosis: > N. asteroides, fever, cough, dyspnea, localized or diffuse pneumonia (symptoms very similar to TBC) If spreads hematogenously => multiple brain abscesses.
- Cutaneous, subcutaneous Nocardiosis: > N. brasiliensis,cellulitis => subcutaneous draining abscess with granules (mycetoma)

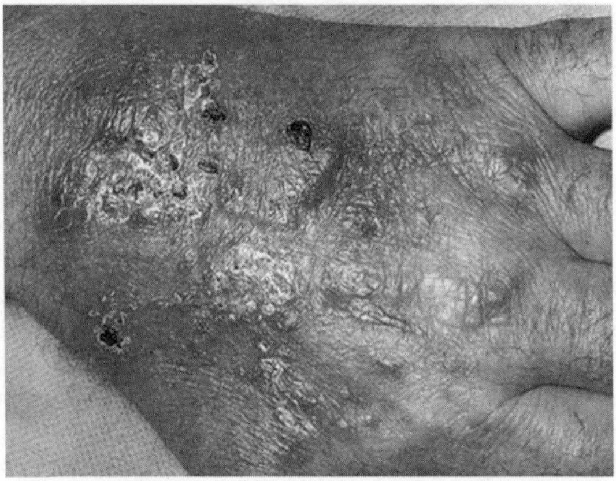

7. **Ans. d. Septicemia** *(Ref: Review of medical microbiology – 13/e p256 Jawetz medical microbiology. 25/e p269)*

Staph. aureus causes many diseases localized and generalized based on its virulence factors. Septicemia is not due to production of toxins

Exfoliatin

- A staphylococcus toxin
- Cleaves the desmosomes in the stratum granulosum
- Separates layers of skin.
- Example: Scalded skin syndrome (occurs more often in infants)

Toxic shock syndrome:

- It is a superantigen, which is a molecule that facilitates the interaction of APCs with T cells

- Instead of this being an antigen-specific interaction (where processed MHC particle is presented on MHC and this is presented to TH cell), superantigen mediates a nonspecific interaction between any T cell and any APC
- This leads to clonal expansion of any T cell that the superantigen helps activate
- This leads to the production of a variety of cytokines and, ultimately, shock
- Staphylococcal enterotoxins are associated with food poisoning too

8. **Ans. a. Heterophile antibody test**

(Ref: Jawetz Medical Microbiology. 25/e p122)

Paul Bunnell test:

- Heterophil antibody tests such as the Paul Bunnell are used in the diagnosis of Infectious mononucleosis
- Heterophil antibodies have the ability to agglutinate red blood cells of different animal species.
- The Paul-Bunnell test uses sheep erythrocytes
- In EBV infection, IgM heterophil antibodies are usually detectable for the first 3 months of infection. They are able to agglutinate sheep erythrocytes; it is absorbed by ox red blood cell but not guinea-pig kidney cells

Description of Paul Bunnel test on positive and negative samples.

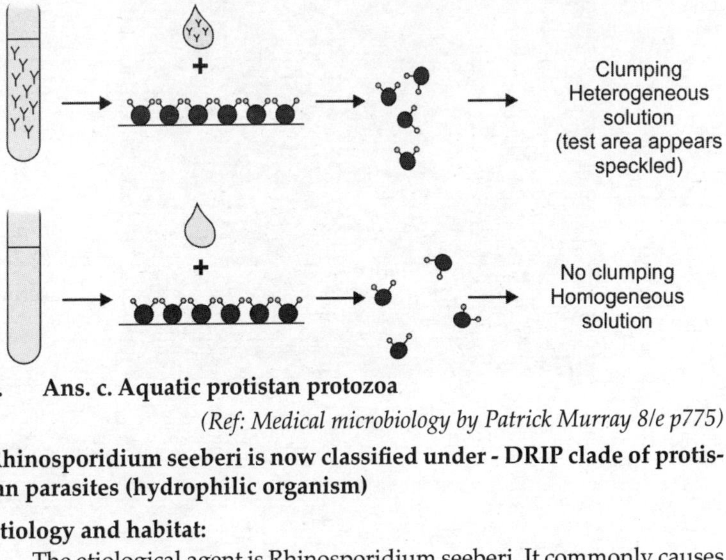

9. **Ans. c. Aquatic protistan protozoa**

(Ref: Medical microbiology by Patrick Murray 8/e p775)

Rhinosporidium seeberi is now classified under - DRIP clade of protistan parasites (hydrophilic organism)

Etiology and habitat:

- The etiological agent is Rhinosporidium seeberi. It commonly causes human infections in India, Sri Lanka, South America, and Africa.

- Its classification has undergone many changes; it was initially thought to be a parasite, then it was considered to be a fungus but now molecular biological techniques have demonstrated that this organism is an aquatic protistan parasite.
- It is currently included in a new class, the Mesomycetozoea

Rhinosporidium life cycle:

- The infection is typically limited to the mucosal epithelium. Its life cycle begins with a round endospore (6-10 μm in diameter), which grows to become a thick-walled sporangium (100-450 μm in diameter) that contains up to several thousand endospores.
- Mature sporangiospores are approximately 7-9 μm in size and escape through a pore that develops in the sporangial wall.

Laboratory diagnosis:

- Nasal secretion (if any) should be collected.
- The entire polyp must be surgically excised; some tissue may be macerated or biopsies are taken.
- The secretions or macerated tissue is observed under microscope with a KOH mount or after staining with H&E.
- Tissue sections can also be stained with GMS or PAS

Rhinosporidium

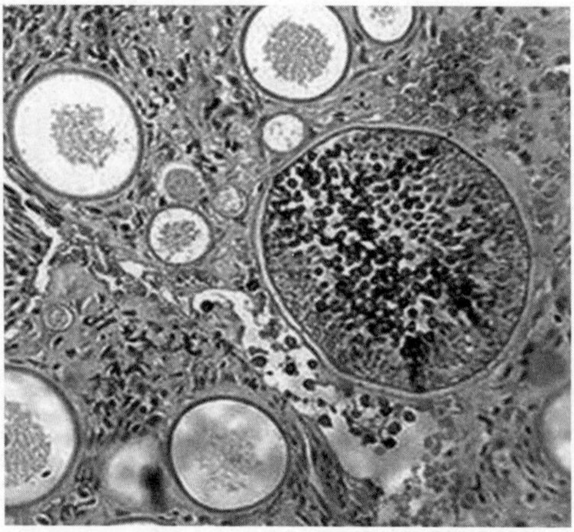

FORENSIC MEDICINE AND TOXICOLOGY

QUESTIONS

1. **A young patient had complaints of acute abdominal pain on and off and tingling sensation of limbs and at times weakness of limbs. She had a history of eating paint from the wall of newly built house. Which of the following enzyme defect will be the cause of her condition?**
   a. ALA dehydratase
   b. ALA synthase
   c. Heme synthase
   d. Coproporphyrin oxidase

2. **Which of the following is not correct regarding teeth features and ethnicity?**
   a. Upper third molar is most commonly absent in Mongolians
   b. In negroes the cusps of molars are wide and deep and shovel shaped cusps in incisors
   c. Caucasians have carabelli cusps
   d. Prominent lingual ridge and labial ridge in Mongols

3. **A young adult came with casualty with history of some substance abuse. His pulse was 130 beats per minute, respiratory rate 30/min, blood gas analysis revealed metabolic acidosis. Urine analysis showed calcium oxalate crystals. Improved on gastric lavage, ethanol, calcium gluconate and 4-methyl pyrazole. What poisoning is it ?**
   a. Ethylene glycol
   b. Methyl alcohol
   c. Formaldehyde
   d. Paraldehyde

4. **Which of the following is correct regarding corporobasal index of sacrum?**
   a. Breadth of 1st sacral vertebra × 100/breadth of 5th lumbar vertebra
   b. Breadth of 5th lumbar vertebra × 100/breadth of all sacral vertebra
   c. Breadth of 5th lumbar vertebra × 100/breadth of base of sacrum
   d. Breadth of 1st sacral vertebra × 100/breadth of base of sacrum

5. **Jack knife position causes death due to:**
   a. Traumatic asphyxia
   b. Burking
   c. Wedging
   d. Positional asphyxia

6. **An adult came to casualty with complaints of rapid heart rate. On examination everythingelse was normal except for episodic tachycardia and occasional extrasystole and amblyopia. Which of the following is the cause of it?**
   a. Nicotine
   b. Cannabis
   c. Atropine
   d. Cocaine

7. **A person was brought to the casualty brought dead and autopsy was performed to find the cause of death. On external examination only finding found was a mark on the chin as in 1st picture. And on internal examination of neck there was the finding on the anterior surface of neck as shown below. Your possible diagnosis is:**

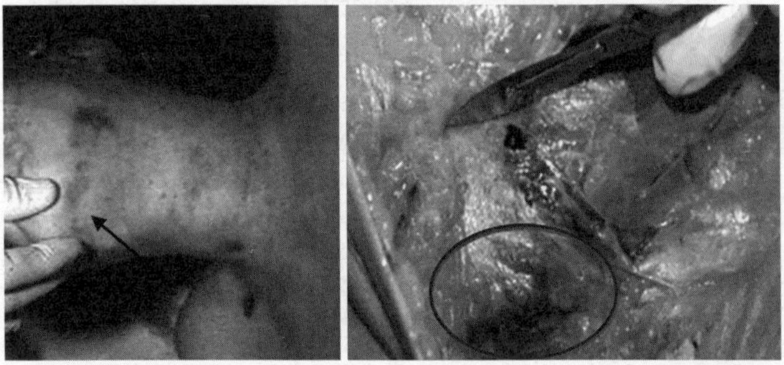

(See Color Plate 8)

   a. Throttling
   b. Strangulation
   c. Mugging
   d. Hanging

EXPLANATIONS

1. Ans. a. ALA dehydratase

(Ref: Principles of Forensic and Toxicology, Rajesh Bardale, 2/e p423)

All clinical features of Lead encephalopathy which is common in children.

Lead poisoning

- Highly toxic substance
- Both adults and children can suffer from the effects of lead poisoning, but childhood — more frequent
- Lead exposure — estimated by measuring levels of lead in the blood (μg/dl)
- Current threshold lead toxicity — 10 μg/dl.

Normal levels of lead

- Less than 20 micrograms/dL of lead in the blood — **Children**
- Less than 5 micrograms/dL of lead in the blood — **Adults**
- Lead inhibits heme synthesis through inhibition of delta ALA–dehydratase, ferrochelatase, porphobilinogen synthase, co-proporphyrinogen oxidase and other enzymes, resulting in the build-up of aminolevulinic acid, coproporphyrins and free erythrocyte protoporphyrin.
- It also inhibits enzyme pyrimidine 5'-nucleotidase, thus increasing erythrocyte fragility.

Management strategies

C/P	Blood Lead Level (μg/dL)	Chelation
Encephalopathy	Any level	BAL + EDTA "high dose"
Symptomatic	> 100	BAL + EDTA "low dose"
Mild symptoms	70-100	Succimer
Asymptomatic	< 70	Medical removal

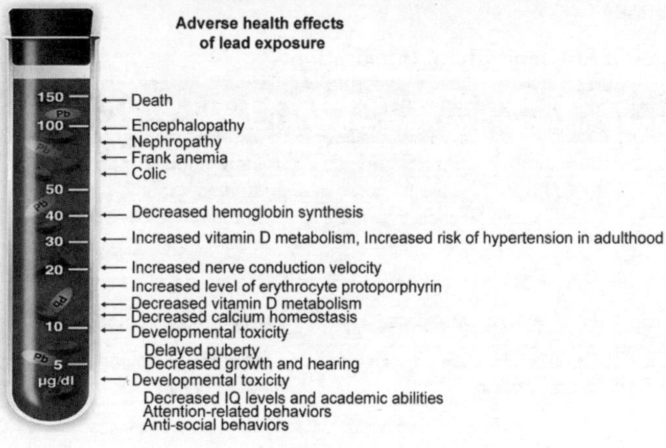

2. **Ans. b. In negroes the cusps of molars are wide and deep and shovel-shaped cusps in incisors**

(Ref: Principles of Forensic and Toxicology, Rajesh Bardale, 2/e p55-59)

- A congenital lack of the third upper molar is most common in Mongoloids
- Shovel-shape incisor teeth has prominent marginal ridges and a deep fossa on their lingual surfaces, which is usually observed in Mongoloid people
- Cusp of Carabelli (a very small fifth cusp or a nodule) on a maxillary 1st molar is present in Caucasoid people.

3. **Ans. a. Ethylene glycol**

(Ref: Principles of Forensic and Toxicology, Rajesh Bardale, 2/e p511)

Ethylene glycol is a colorless, odorless, sweet-tasting chemical. It is poisonous if swallowed. Ethylene glycol is a central nervous system (CNS) depressant that can produce acute effects similar to those of ethanol. These CNS effects predominate during the first hours after exposure.

MOA – The main toxicity results from hepatic metabolism of ethylene glycol to glycoaldehyde, glycolate, glyoxylate, and oxalate. These metabolites inhibit:

- Oxidative phosphorylation and cellular respiration
- Glucose and serotonin metabolism
- Protein synthesis
- DNA replication
- Ribosomal RNA formation.

The accumulation of organic acid metabolites, especially glycolic acid, results in anion gap metabolic acidosis which affects many cellular functions.

Stages of Ethylene Glycol Intoxication

Stage	Onset after ingestion	Primary systems affected	Signs and symptoms
1	30 minutes to 12 hours	Central nervous system	Inebriation, euphoria, ataxia, slurred speech, drowsiness, irritation, restlessness, and disorientation
		Gastrointestinal	Nausea and vomiting
		Metabolic	Elevated osmolar gap
2	12 to 24 hours	Cardiovascular	Mild hypertension, tachycardia, and shock

Contd...

Contd...

Stage	Onset after ingestion	Primary systems affected	Signs and symptoms
		Pulmonary	Tachypnea, adult respiratory distress symdrome, pulmonary edema, and pneumonitis
		Metabolic	Metabolic acidosis with elevated anion gap and decreased osmolar gap, possible tetany from hypocalcemia, and hyperventilation
3	24 to 72 hours	Renal	Flank pain, costovertebral angle tenderness, oliguric renal failure, hyperkalemia, and hypocalcemia
		Metabolic	May have normal anion and osmolal gaps.

(Note: Metabolic acidosis also seen with methanol but calcium oxalate crystals with renal failure are characteristic of Ethylene glycol).

4. **Ans. d. Breadth of 1st sacral vertebra × 100/breadth of base of sacrum**

(Ref: Principles of Forensic and Toxicology, Rajesh Bardale, 2/e p111)

- Corporo-basal (CB) index is a sex differentiating index used for sacrum

Corporo-Basal Index =	Breadth of body of 1st sacral vertebra / Breadth of base of sacrum	× 100

Corporo-basal index: (Transverse diameter of body of S1 × 100)/ Width of sacrum

- It is > 42 in Males and < 42 in females
- CB index is more in male (cf. with other indices)

Other indices for determination of sex from skeletal remains are:
Washburn or ischiopubic index for hip bone (73–94 in males, 91–115 in females)
Sacral index for sacrum (<114 in males, >114 in females)
Sternal index for sternum (46.2 in males, 54.3 in females)

5. **Ans. d. Positional asphyxia**

(Ref: Principles of Forensic and Toxicology, Rajesh Bardale. 2/e p285)

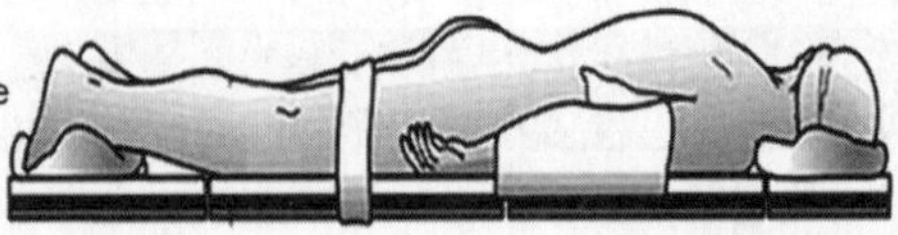

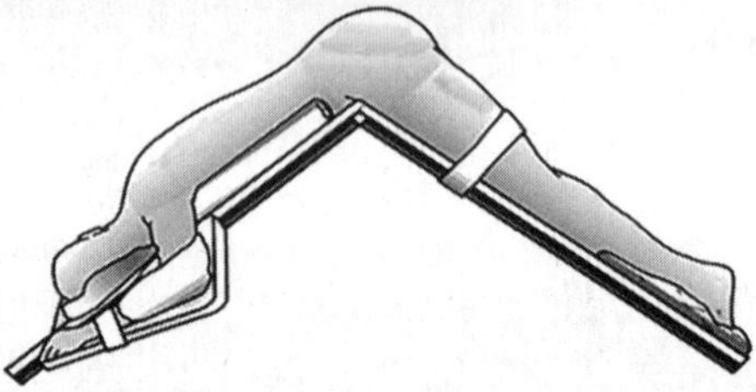

- (Jack knife position is, where the chest is bent /pressed to the knee. This causes physiologic alteration in the relationship between the diaphragm and the lungs. The level of the lungs go below the level of the diaphragm. Lungs cant operate to its optimal best and the person eventually succumb to asphyxia.)

6. **Ans. a. Nicotine**

(Ref: KSN Reddy; Essential of FMT, 33/e p615/ Krishan Vij, TB of FMT, 5/e p526)

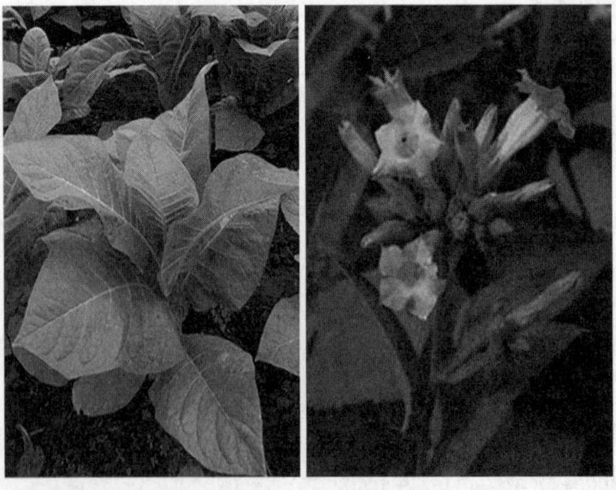

Actions of tobacco

- Chemical reactions in the nerve endings which increases heart rate, memory, alertness and reaction time.
- Neurotransmitters called dopamine and later endorphins are released in the brain producing feelings of pleasure and satisfaction.

- As an addictive drug, nicotine has two very potent issues—it is a stimulant as well as depressant.
- **Effects of Nicotine – PNS and CNS Communication**
  - Adrenal glands in PNS affect CNS
  - Nicotine stimulates release of epinephrine
  - Causes CNS arousal and decrease in alpha activity.
- **Brainstem Centers**
  - Reticular activating system
  - Direct stimulation causes arousal
  - Widespread cholinergic projections`1`.3
  - Substantial nigra, basal forebrain, thalamus, and cerebellum.

Medullary Respiratory Centers

- Direct and indirect stimulation
  - Overdose of nicotine
  - Blocking of these centers and neuromuscular junctions
  - Respiratory arrest
  - **Cardiac irritability marked by irregular action, palpitation, and sometimes pain, believed to occur as a result of the heavy use of tobacco** is also known as tobacco heart.

7. **Ans. a. Throttling**

(Ref: Principles of Forensic and Toxicology, Rajesh Bardale, 2/e p299)

It is always homicidal. At times however, a mild playful tweak on the neck has resulted in death from vagal inhibition.

- Signs of asphyxia are seen. In addition, the following specific findings may be present.
- Bruising of the neck.
- Occurs due to the assailant's fingers grasping the neck.
- Usually circular, dark red or purple in color, and are 1-2 cm in size.
- If the fingers slide over the skin, elongated marks may be seen.
- Abrasions on the neck.
- Scratches may be caused by the fingernails of either the assailant or the victim.
- Curved or linear.
- During autopsy, scrapings from under the fingernails of the deceased may be taken for DNA fingerprinting and compared with that of the suspect, because the victim may have scratched the assailant in an attempt to ward off the attack.

Internal appearances:

- Tissues of the neck are often markedly contused.
- Bleeding may be seen in the strap muscles or platysma.
- If excessive force has been applied, bleeding from larynx may have occurred.

ORTHOPEDICS

QUESTIONS

1. **March fracture in metatarsal following stress is seen in ______ of second metatarsal:**
   a. Head
   b. Neck
   c. Shaft
   d. Base

2. **In polio paralysis; hand, knee gait due to weakness of:**
   a. Gluteus maximus
   b. Gluteus medius
   c. Quadriceps
   d. Gastroc-soleus

3. **A 4-year-old boy fell on outstretched hand, X-ray is as shown below. Which of the following vessel is most commonly affected?**

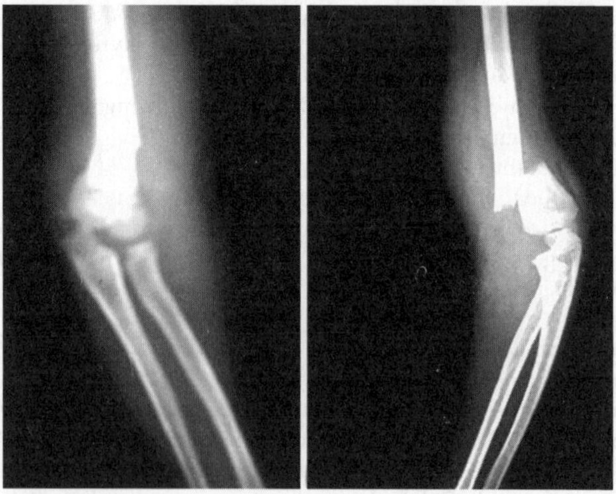

   a. Ulnar artery
   b. Radial artery
   c. Brachial artery
   d. Cubital vein

4. **An elderly patient slipped in bathroom and sustained injury over hip. X-ray is shown below. Her attitude of leg will be:**

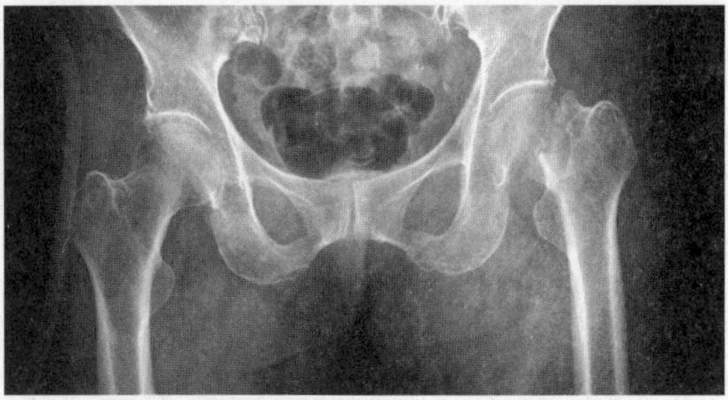

a. Shortened abducted and externally rotated
b. Shortened and abducted
c. Lengthened and internally rotated
d. Flexed and adducted and internally rotated

5. Which of the position is being tested in the picture given below?

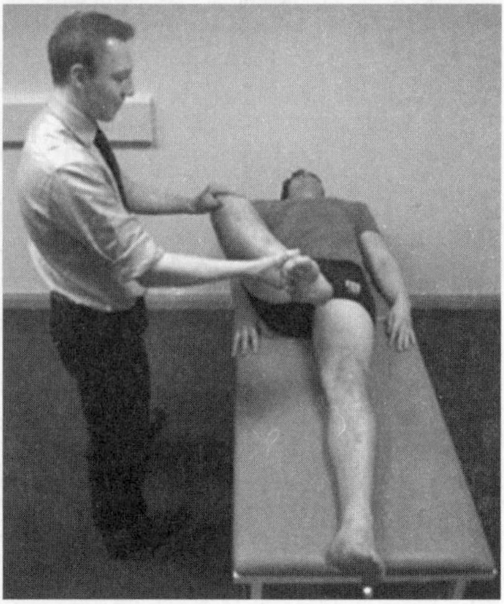

a. Internal rotation
b. External rotation
c. Abduction
d. Flexion

6. Which of the following is the most common squeal of traumatic dislocation of shoulder?

a. Normal shoulder healing and normal movements
b. Recurrent dislocation of shoulder
c. Rotator cuff injury
d. Subcapsular tendonitis

7. **Which of the following is true regarding Galeazzi fracture dislocation?**
   a. Interosseous membrane tear with ulnar shaft fracture
   b. Radial collateral ligament tear with interosseous membrane tear with radial shaft fracture
   c. Interosseous membrane tear with triangular fibrocartilage complex (TFCC) tear and ulnar shaft fracture
   d. Interosseous membrane tear with triangular fibrocartilage complex (TFCC) tear and radial shaft fracture

8. **A patient came with complaints of inability to move his 4th and 5th digit, cannot hold pen and he was not able to hold paper between fingers. Which of the following site given below is the probable cause of injury to the nerve in question?**

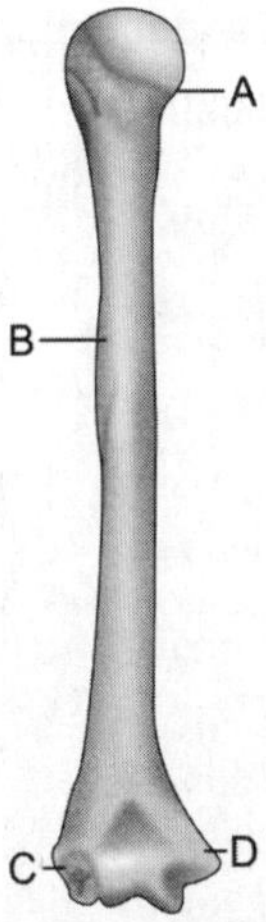

   a. A b. B
   c. C d. D

9. **What is the best management for fracture of patella shown in the image?**

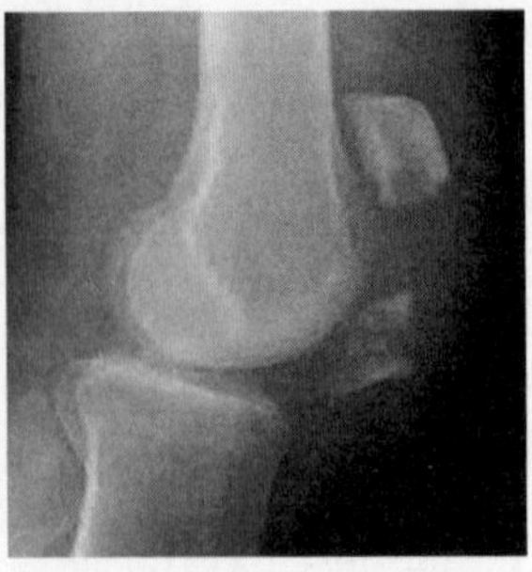

a. Intramedullary nail
b. Tension band wiring
c. Patellectomy
d. Above Knee cast

10. **Which of the following is bone holding forceps used in orthopedic surgeries?**

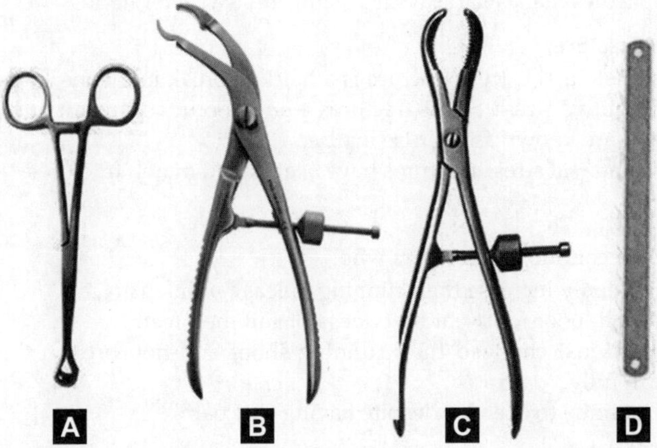

a. A
b. B
c. C
d. D

11. **Haglund deformity is seen in which of the following joints?**
a. Knee
b. Wrist
c. Elbow
d. Ankle

12. **The growth of cartilage following fracture will be increased by which of the following?**
a. Intramedullary nail
b. K-wire fixation
c. Strict immobilization
d. Repeated tiny movements at the fracture sit

EXPLANATIONS

1. Ans. b. Neck

(Ref. Campbell's Operative Orthopaedics, 12/e p2676)

Going by Cambells orthopaedics. Answers is Neck. Textbook of orthopaedics maheswari says it's shaft, still we prefer neck.

Stress fracture:

- A metatarsal stress fracture is a hairline break in a bone, caused by repetitive stress. Stress fractures tend to occur as a result of overuse and are known as overuse injuries.
- Metatarsal stress fractures have been called march fractures.

Cause:

They are common in runners who:

- Suddenly increase their running mileage or intensity.
- Run in poor footwear that does not suit their feet.
- Have just changed their running shoes and not 'broken them in' carefully.
- Continue to exercise despite having foot pain.

Complications:

- A fracture of the first metatarsal bone can lead to later arthritis of the big toe joint.
- A fracture at the base of the fifth metatarsal bone is often mistaken for an ankle sprain. This would usually result in it not being rested or supported enough. This could lead to problems in healing and continuing pain.

2. Ans. c. Quadriceps *(Ref: Textbook of Orthopaedics. Kulkarni, p567)*

Poliomyelitis

- In poliomyelitis; hand to knee gait is the sum of quadriceps weakness and fixed knee flexion deformity.

Types of gait:

- Hypokinetic gait/shuffling gait/festinating gait—Parkinson
- Spastic gait: UMN lesion.
- Antalgic gait: Tarsal tunnel syndrome or any joint pain.
- En-bloc gait: Vestibular ataxia (also may be cerebellar ataxia)
- High-steppage gait: Common peroneal injury
- Waddling gait: Duchene muscular dystrophy.
- Staggering gait: Alcoholics, Friedrich's ataxia
- Scissoring gait: Cerebral palsy.
- Magnetic gait: Hydrocephalus.

3. Ans. c. Brachial artery

(Ref. Rockwood & Green's Fractures in Children, 6/e Chapter 14)

- Injury to the brachial artery: This is a complication commonly associated with a displaced supracondylar fracture. The brachial artery is usually injured by the sharp edge of the proximal fragment.

In case of vascular injury the below is the protocol given for management:

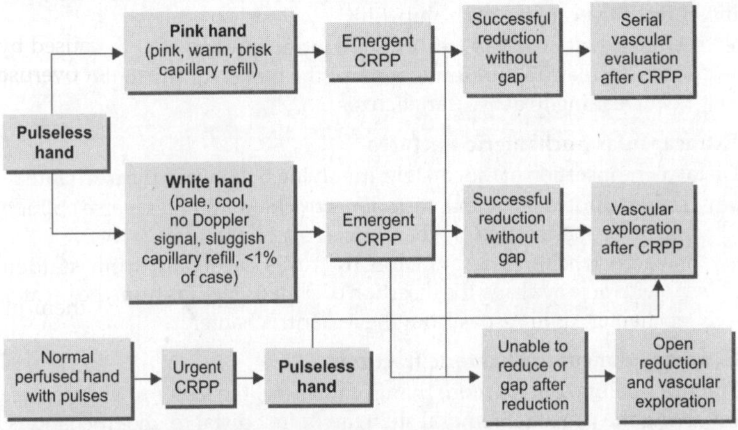

Garland classification and treatment compiled:

Type I	Nondisplaced, beware of subtle medial comminution leading to cubitus varus Anterior periosteum detached from anterior humerus by up to 3 cm (but not torn) Treated with cast immobilization x 3–4 wks, with radiographs at 1 wk, pull pins at 3 wks
Type II	Displaced, posterior cortex and posterior periosteal hinge intact IIA - no rotational deformity/fragment translation IIB - has rotational deformity/fragment translation (high risk of coronal/rotational malalignment) Treated with CRPP
Type III	Completely displaced, no cortical contact but has intact posterior periosteal hinge Treated with CRPP
Type IV	Complete periosteal disruption with instability in flexion and extension Treated with CRPP
Medial comminution in Type II	Collapse of medial column, loss of Baumann angle (leads to varus malunion/classic gunstock deformity) Treated with CRPP
Flexion type	Shear mechanism, oblique orientation, inherently unstable Treated with CRPP

4. Ans. a. Shortened abducted and externally rotated

(Ref: Campbell's Operative Orthopaedics 12/e Vol 4, p20-23)

"The physical examination typically reveals an extremity that is shortened and externally rotated."

Classification of neck of femur fracture:

Intracapsular fractures

Involve the femoral neck between the edge of the femoral head and insertion of the capsule of the hip joint.

- Around half of all hip fractures are intracapsular.
- Intracapsular fractures may disrupt the blood supply to the femoral head, leading to avascular necrosis.

Extracapsular trochanteric fractures

Distal to the insertion of the capsule, involving or between the trochanters.

- They include intertrochanteric or pertrochanteric and reverse oblique fractures and isolated trochanteric avulsion fractures.
- Isolated trochanteric avulsion fractures can result from sudden violent force avulsing the insertion of gluteus medius from the greater trochanter, or iliopsoas from the lesser trochanter.

Extracapsular subtrochanteric fractures

Fractures below, but no more than 5 cm below, the lesser trochanter, i.e. involving the proximal femoral shaft, at, or just distal to, the trochanters

Intracapsular neck of femur classification:

- Garden I: Trabeculae angulated, inferior cortex intact. No significant displacement.
- Garden II: Trabeculae in line but a fracture line is visible from superior to inferior cortex. No significant displacement.
- Garden III: Obvious complete fracture line with slight displacement and/or rotation of the femoral head.
- **Garden IV: Gross, often complete, displacement of the femoral head.**

5. Ans. b. External rotation

This is a simple question to assess the examination skills of a medical graduate.

Few examination that can be asked in relation to hip joint:

- FABER Test
  - Flexion Abduction External Rotation
  - Also known as Patrick's Test or Figure of Four Test
- FADIR Test
  - Flexion Adduction Internal Rotation
- Ober Test
  - Passive Hip Adduction
- Log Roll Test (Freiberg Test)
  - Passive Supine Hip Rotation (with hip and knee extended)

- Stinchfield Test
  - Straight Leg Raise Against Resistance

Faber:

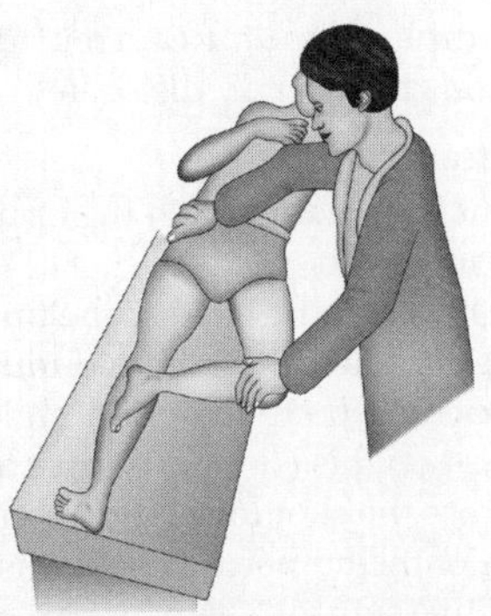

FADIR:

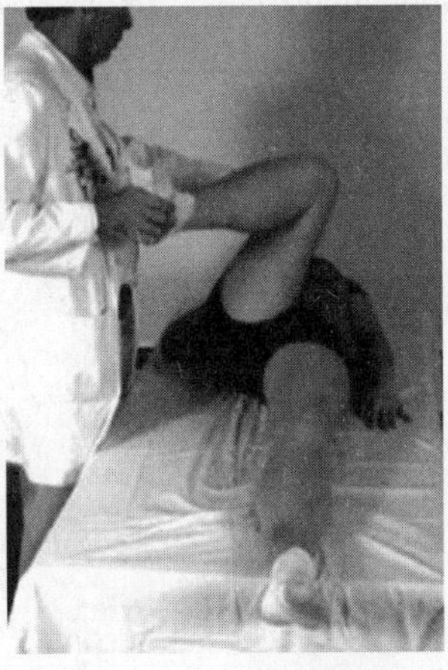

Ober test:

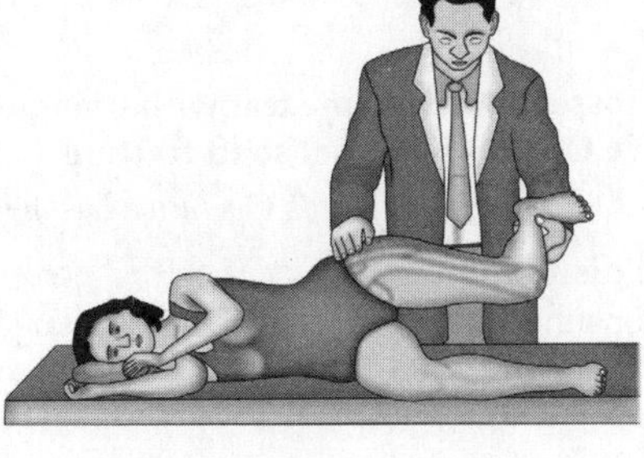

6. **Ans. b. Recurrent dislocation of shoulder**

(Ref: Campbell's Operative Orthopaedics 12/e p24030)

Dislocation of shoulder and squeal:

- Most common complication is Recurrent dislocation (50% of all shoulder dislocations recurrently dislocate)

Tests for sholder dislocation:

- **Duga's test:** Patient is asked to touch the opposite shoulder. Unable to do so, test is positive.
- **Hamilton ruler test:** When the head of the humerus is in the glenoid cavity, the bulging contour of the deltoid muscle prevents one from placing a ruler touching both acromion and lateral condyle of the humerus. In dislocation this contour is lost and it is possible to place a ruler straight across the shoulder touching both, the acromion and the lateral condyle of the humerus. The test is said to be positive.
- **Bryant's sign:** Positive sign is shown by lowering and prominence of the anterior axillary fold.
- **Callaway's test/sign:** Increase in girth of the shoulder

Kocher method of shoulder dislocation:

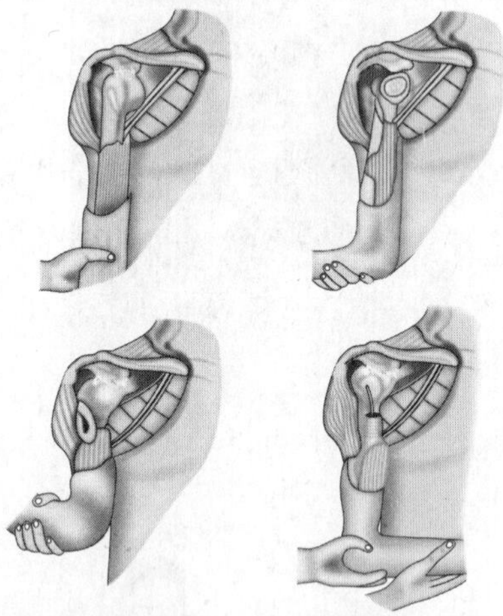

7. **Ans. d. Interosseous membrane tear with triangular fibrocartilage complex (TFCC) tear and radial shaft fracture**

(Ref: Campbell's Operative Orthopaedics 12/e p1385)

Galeazzi fracture dislocation:

- "Dislocation or subluxation of the distal radio-ulnar joint in association with a solitary fracture of the radius at the junction of the middle and distal third"

- "Fracture of the lower third of the radius with dislocation or subluxation of the distal radioulnar joint."
- "Distal radioulnar joint (DRUJ) injury"

Classification	Description	Notes
Type 1	Radial fracture <7.5 cm from distal articular surface	Higher incidence of DRUJ instability
Type 2	Radial fracture >7.5 cm from distal articular surface	

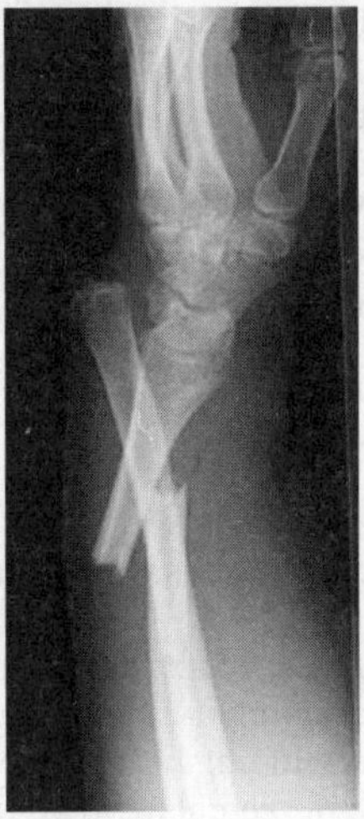

8. **Ans. d. D**

(Ref. Essential Orthopaedics - J. Maheshwari, Chapter 10; Campbell's Operative Orthopaedics 12/e – Chapter 62, 68)

The most probable nerve injured in this case is ULNAR nerve.

Ulnar Nerve – Sites of Entrapment

- At the elbow
  - Arcade of Struthers—Myofascial band extending from medial intermuscular septum to the medial head of triceps, 8 cm above medial epicondyle
  - Medial intermuscular septum where it pierces
  - Medial head of triceps
  - Medial epicondyle
  - Epicondylar groove
  - Cubital tunnel between 2 heads of FCU which are connected by aponeurotic Osborne's ligament
  - Flexor pronator aponeurosis between FDP and FDS.

- At the Guyon's canal
  - Zone I: Proximal to bifurcation
  - Zone II: Distal to bifurcation. Contains deep branch.
  - Zone III: Contains the superficial branch
- Functional losses in ulnar nerve injury
  - Loss of key pinch due to paralysis of adductor pollicis and first dorsal Interossei.
  - Clawing due to paralysis of Interossei and lumbricals in presence of functioning extrinsic extensors leading to MCPJ hyperextension and functioning long flexors leading to flexion of IPJ.
  - Loss of forward flexion of mobile fourth and fifth carpometacarpal joints lead to loss of transverse palmar arch manifested as inability to cup the hand to hold water.
  - Loss of normal integrated MCPJ and IPJ flexion. Normal finger flexion starts at MCPJ followed by IPJ. In ulnar nerve palsy IPJ flexes first followed by MCPJ. This rolling motion will lead to inability to grasp objects.
  - Loss of FDP function of medial 2 digits in high ulnar nerve palsy leads to diminished grip strength.

Clinical signs:

- Duchenne sign: Clawing
- Cross finger test: Inability to cross index and middle finger over each other.
- Pitres-Testut sign: Inability to abduct middle finger to either side.
- Wartenberg sign: Abduction of little finger.
- Loss of normal sequence of finger flexion: Normally MCPJ flexes then the IPJ flexes. In ulnar nerve palsy MCPJ flexes last.
- Loss of key pinch
- Jeannes sign: MCPJ of thumb hyperextended during key pinch.
- Masse sign: Loss of hypothenar eminence and flattened palmar metacarpal arch.
- Pollock sign: Inability to flex DIPJ of little and ring fingers.
- Froments sign: Substitution of adductor pollicis by FPL during key pinch.

9. **Ans. b. Tension band wiring**

(Ref. Campbell's Operative Orthopaedics 12/e – Chapter 452)

- Transverse fractures
  - The patella can be split transversely by indirect violence, e.g. a sudden violent contraction of the quadriceps, gives rise to a fracture with the fracture line running transversely across the patella, dividing it into two. These injuries split not only the patella but also the quadriceps expansions on either side.
  - Left untreated, the fragments separate widely and quadriceps function is lost.

- Treatment
  - Internal fixation is required. A **TENSION BAND WIRE** is usually adequate.

Comminuted fractures

- The patella is fractured by a blow directly to the knee, often in a road traffic accident
- Treatment - **PATELLECTOMY**

10. Ans. b. B

This is again to test the clinical acumen of MBBS graduate.

Naming of the instruments above:

- A- Babcock Forceps
- B- Bone Holding Forceps
- C- Reduction Forceps
- D- Hack Saw Blade

11. Ans. d. Ankle *(Ref: Campbell's Operative Orthopaedics 12/e p3963)*

Haglund deformity (pump bump) and retrocalcaneal bursitis

- Haglund deformity (also known as a pump bump or Bauer bump or Mulhulland deformity) is defined as bony enlargement formed at posterosuperior aspect of calcaneum
- Haglund's deformity can be related to rigid back (counter) of pump style shoes, giving it the name "pump bump."
- Shoes with a rigid counter can increase the pressure at the posterior calcaneus creating an irritation that aggravates the bone enlargement.
- The most important criteria for the evaluation of the biomechanical patterns of the deformity are the posterior calcaneal angle and the pitch angle (calcaneal inclination angle).
- Women aged 20 to 30 years are often affected due to the use of high heeled shoes.

Treatment: Non-surgical treatment involves biomechanical, physical and pharmacologic therapies. Surgery very rarely performed for extremes of cases.

- Rest and sometimes immobilization can help to reduce the inflammation
- Ice: Indicated to reduce swelling.
- Medication: Oral nonsteroidal anti-inflammatory drugs (NSAIDs).
- Stretching exercises: Help to relieve tension from the Achilles tendon.
- Shoe modification: Decrease heel counter to reduce pressure on the Achilles tendon
- Physical therapy: Ultrasounds, laser therapy, tecar therapy
- Orthotic devices: Indicated to support the arch and to decrease the Achilles tendon tension

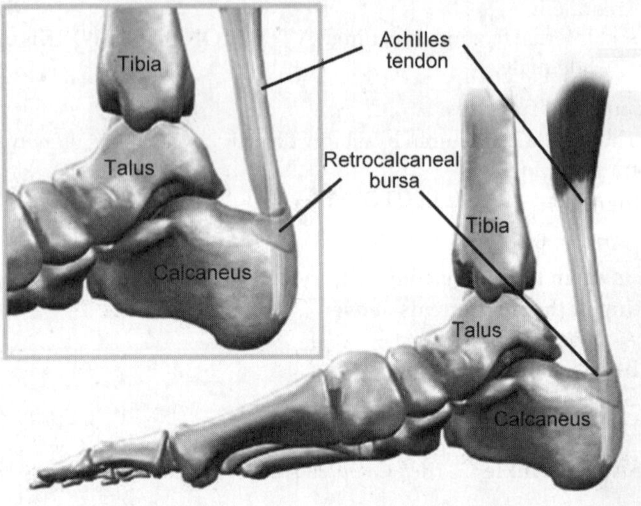

12. **Ans. d. Repeated tiny movements at the fracture site**

(Ref: Mercer's Textbook of Orthopaedics and Trauma, 10/e, Chapter 19, p270)

Repeat from last AIIMS exam.

The mechanical stability of the fracture site influences the repair process.

Factors affecting fracture healing:

- Blood supply
  - Soft tissue injury
  - Radiation
  - Chemical or thermal burns
  - Infection
  - Anemia and hypoxia
  - Denervation
  - Excessive compression (more than 30 lbs)
  - Age
- Excessive movement
  - Inadequate immobilisation
  - Inadequate fixation or compliance
- Gap
  - Intact fellow bone
  - Interposed soft tissue
  - Distraction of bones
- Other
  - Nutrition (Vit C required for normal collagen)
  - Drugs (corticosteriods inhibit osteoblast differentiation)

OPHTHALMOLOGY

QUESTIONS

1. **Identify the test shown below:**

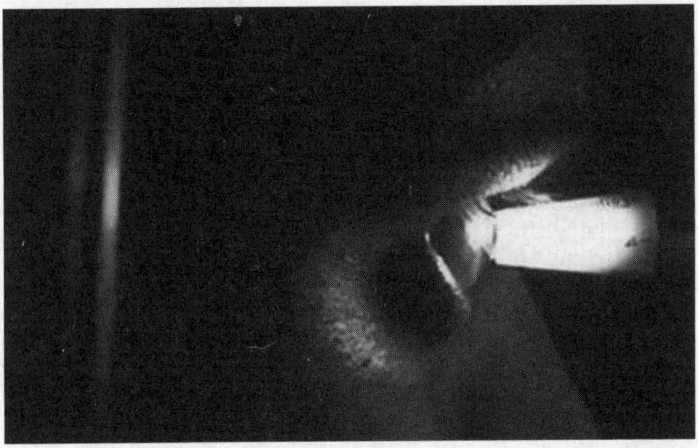

(See Color Plate 9)

   a. Tonometry
   b. Laser interferometry
   c. Pachymetry
   d. Refractometer

2. **A 60-year-old with cataract surgery, post 1 year came with complaints of diminished vision. And shows the following finding. Diagnosis:**

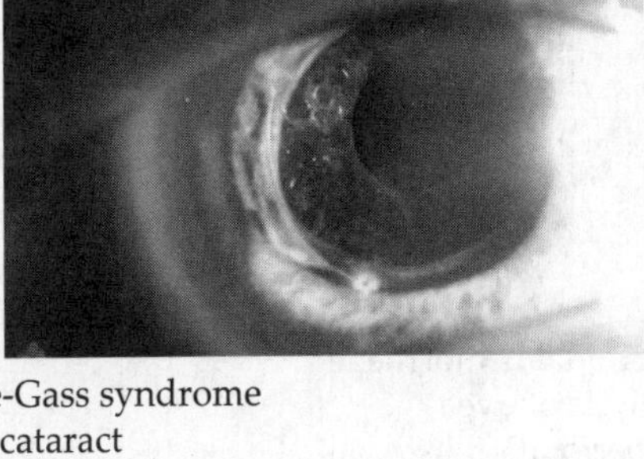

(See Color Plate 9)

   a. Irvine-Gass syndrome
   b. After cataract
   c. UGH syndrome

d. Endophthalmitis

3. **"Silent choroid" on FFA is feature of:**
   a. Best's disease
   b. Age related macular degeneration
   c. Stargardt's disease
   d. Cystoid macular edema

4. **Identify the below finding:**

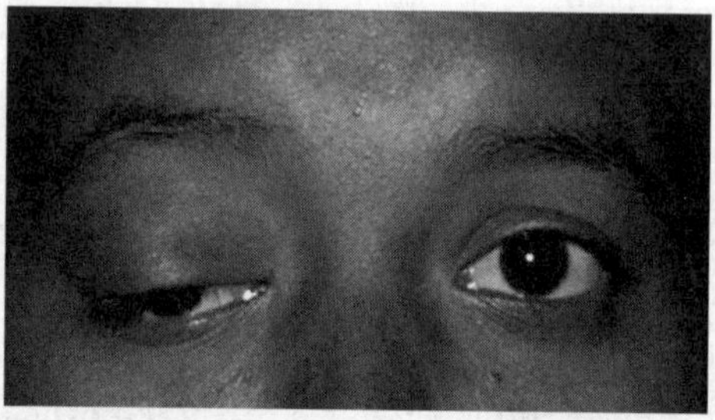

(See Color Plate 9)

   a. Ptosis of right eye
   b. Entropion of right eye
   c. Lagophthalmos right eye
   d. Ectropion left eye

5. **Visual pathway defect at the level of optic chiasma will result in:**
   a. Binasal hemianopia
   b. Bitemporal hemianopia
   c. Central scotoma
   d. Bilateral hemianopia

6. **The following picture shows—(1) abrasion, (2) corneal ulcer, (3) corneal perforation and foreign body. Which of the following will not cause hypotonic maculopathy?**

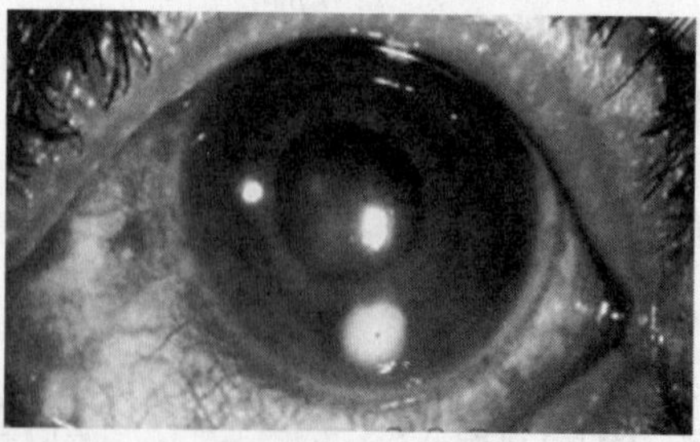

(See Color Plate 10)

   a. Suprachoroidal hemorrhage
   b. Cyclodialysis of uvea
   c. Corneal perforation
   d. Filtration site leak

EXPLANATIONS

1. **Ans. a. Tonometry**

(Ref: AK Khurana Comprehensive Ophthalmology 6/e p510-511)

- Picture shows measurement of Intraocular pressure **(Tonometry)** with Goldmann tonometer

Types of tonometer

- **Tonopen and Mackay Marg** tonometers are used in **irregular corneas.**
- **Maklakov tonometer** is an applanation tonometer with **variable applanation area and fixed force.**

Laser Interferometry:

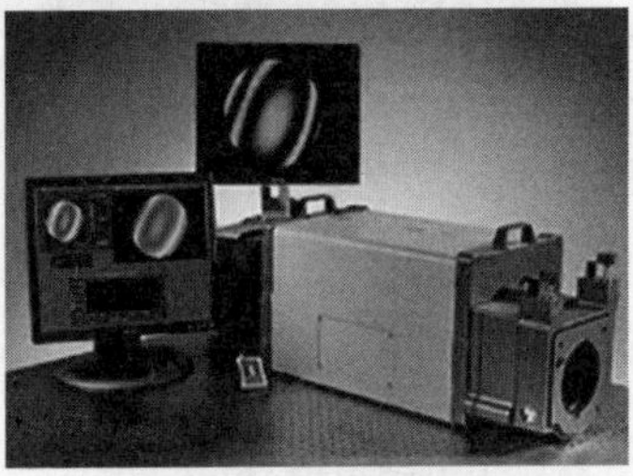

Corneal Pachymetry:

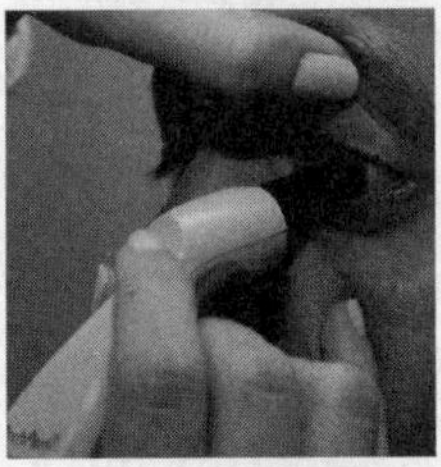

Refractometer:

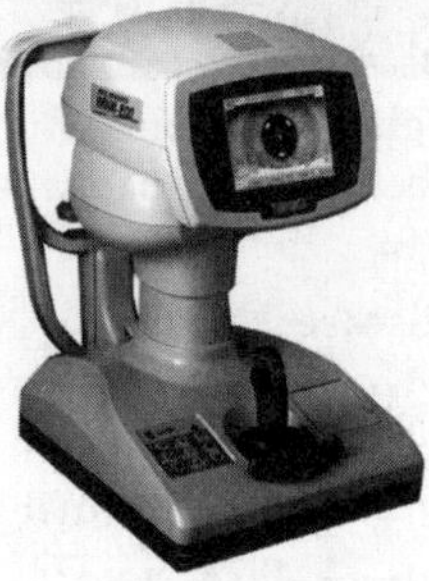

2. **Ans. b. After cataract**

(Ref: A.K.Khurana Comprehensive Ophthalmology 6/e p215)

- The picture shows **"Elsching pearls"** one of the common type of after cataract
  - **Soemmering ring**: whitish annular or doughnut-shaped proliferation of residual cells that classically formed almost in the periphery of the capsular bag

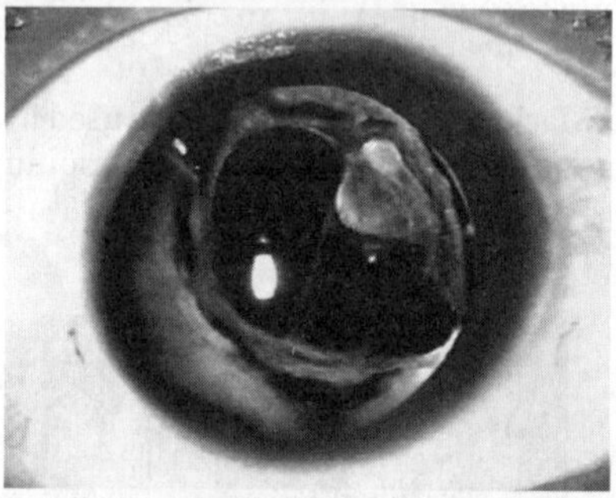

Soemmering ring

- Treatment of after cataract: Capsulotomy using **Nd:YAG laser**
- **Irvine-Gass syndrome** is the term used for cystoid macular edema (CME) after cataract surgery

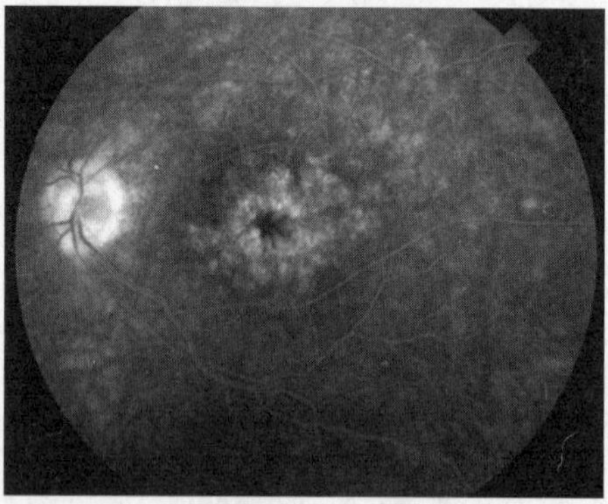

- UGH Syndrome: **Uveitis-Glaucoma-Hyphema Syndrome** occurs when there is contact between lens haptics and uveal tissue or corneal endothelium is present.

3. **Ans. c. Stargardt's disease**

(Ref: Kanski's Clinical Ophthalmology 8/e p233)

Stargardt's disease is also called Stargardt macular dystrophy, juvenile macular degeneration, or fundus flavimaculatus.

The disease causes progressive damage—or degeneration—of the macula, which is a small area in the center of the retina that is responsible for sharp, straight-ahead vision

- Stargardt's disease: About 80% cases show silent choroid in early stage
- Most common macular dystrophy

Inheritance: Autosomal recessive trait very common typical form (STGD1) caused by mutations involving the ***ABCA4 gene*** maps to the short arm of **chromosome 1 (1p22.1)**

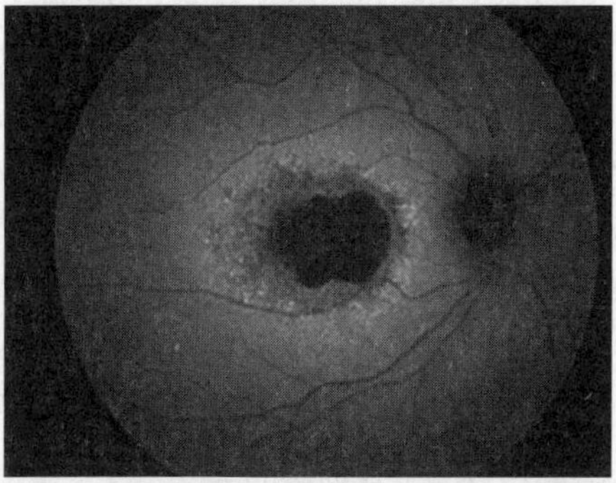

FFA → D**ark/ silent** choroid due to blocking of choroidal fluorescence and **bull's-eye pattern of macular transmission defect**.

4. Ans. a. Ptosis of right eye

(Ref: AK Khurana Comprehensive Ophthalmology 6/e p379)

- Picture shows drooping of right eye upper lid which is called **ptosis** surgical treatment for various types of ptosis are.

Ptosis surgery	Requisite levator action	Amount of ptosis that can be treated	Indications
Fasanella servat	Good	< 2 mm	Horner's syndrome
Levator resection Anterior approach (Everbuch's)	Moderate	Any	Larger resection in congenital and acquired ptosis
Levator resection Conjunctival approach (Blaskovic's)	Moderate	Any	Moderate con-genital or acquired ptosis
Levator resection with aponeurotic reinsertion	Moderate	Any	Acquired ptosis
Frontalis suspension	Poor	> 2 mm	Congenital espe-cially parcuss gun or for temporary relief

5. **Ans. b. Bitemporal hemianopia**

(Ref: Kanski's Clinical Ophthalmology 8/e p820)

Visual Pathway:

- Visual pathway may be summerized as:
  - Optic nerve→optic chisma→optic radiation → optic tract → lateral geniculate body→ optic radiation →occipital lobe
  - Beyond the optic tract, the fibres pass through the lateral geniculate body and the optic radiation. The inferior fibres of the optic radiation pass through temporal lobe (Mayer's Loop), whereas the superior fibres pass through parietal lobe.
  - Lesion at the optic chiasma most commonly causes **bitemporal hemianopia**.
  - The most common lesions producing the chiasmal syndrome include:
    - Pituitary adenoma
    - Parasellar meningioma
    - Craniopharyngioma
    - Parasellar internal carotid artery aneurysm

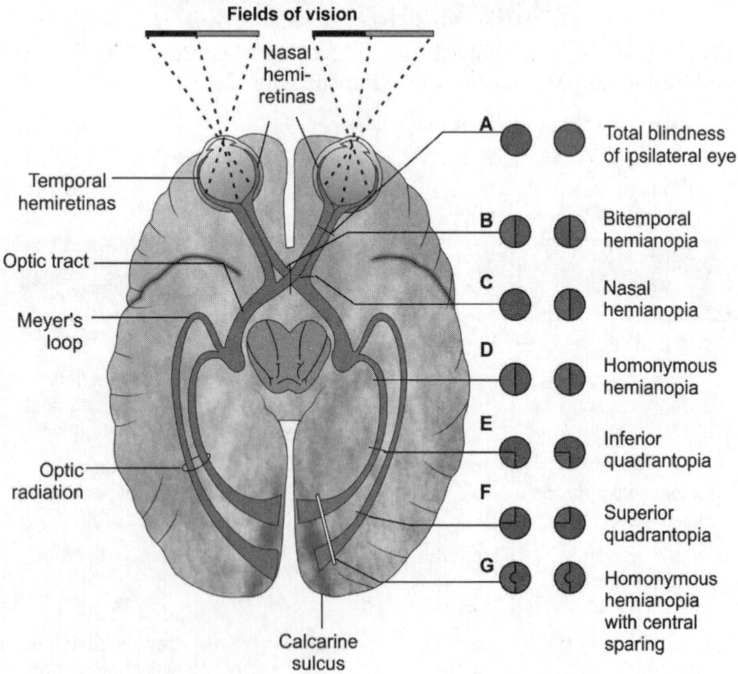

6. **Ans. a. Suprachoroidal hemorrhage**

(Ref: Kanski's Clinical Ophthalmology 8/e p637)

➤ Causes of hypotonic maculopathy

Postoperative hypotony	Traumatic hypotony	Bilateral hypotony	Miscellaneous forms of hypotony
❍ Overfiltration ❍ **Bleb leak** ❍ Wound leak ❍ Iridocyclitis ❍ Cyclodialysis ❍ Ciliochoroidal detachment ❍ Retinal detachment	❍ **Scleral /corneal perforation** ❍ Retinal detachment ❍ **Cyclodialysis** ❍ Iridocyclitis ❍ Ciliochoroidal detachment	❍ Osmotic dehydration ❍ Diabetic coma ❍ Uremia ❍ Myotonic dystrophy	❍ Ciliary body hypoperfusion from vascular occlusive disease

ENT

QUESTIONS

1. **The audiogram shown below gives following diagnosis:**

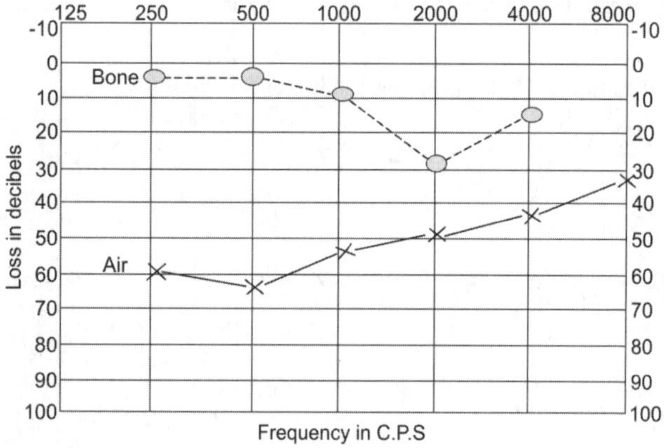

a. Otosclerosis
b. Ototoxicity
c. Meniere disease
d. Noise induced hearing loss

2. **A 6-year-old develops gradual progressive hoarseness of voice over three months and respiratory distress for 2 weeks. Diagnosis is:**

a. Croup
b. Acute epigloittis
c. Vocal nodule
d. Respiratory papillomatosis

3. **Identify the following line shown in the below picture:**

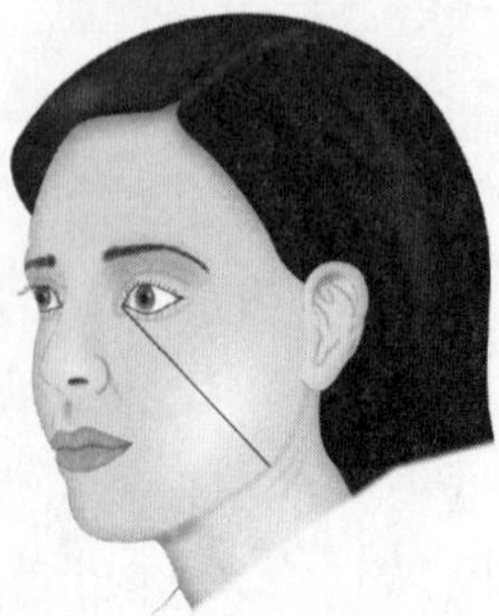

a. Ohngren's line
b. Kassum's line
c. Donaldson's line
d. Frankfurt's line

4. **Which of the following is not ligated in case of epistaxis control?**

a. Anterior ethmoidal artery
b. Maxillary artery
c. External carotid artery
d. Internal carotid artery

EXPLANATIONS

1. Ans. a. Otosclerosis

(Ref: PL Dhingra 6/e p29)

This audiogram shows conductive pattern of hearing loss

- For CONDUCTIVE hearing loss
  - Air-Bone gap present and BC > AC
- (i.e. BC should be in the normal range, AC should be in the hearing loss range
- For SENSORINEURAL hearing loss:
  - No A-B gap
- Both AC and BC should be in hearing loss range (i.e. > 25 db in audiometry)

So, Answer is Option a. Otoslerosis

- **CARHART'S notch,** a dip in bone conduction at 2,000 Hz is seen.
- Disappears after successful stapes surgery

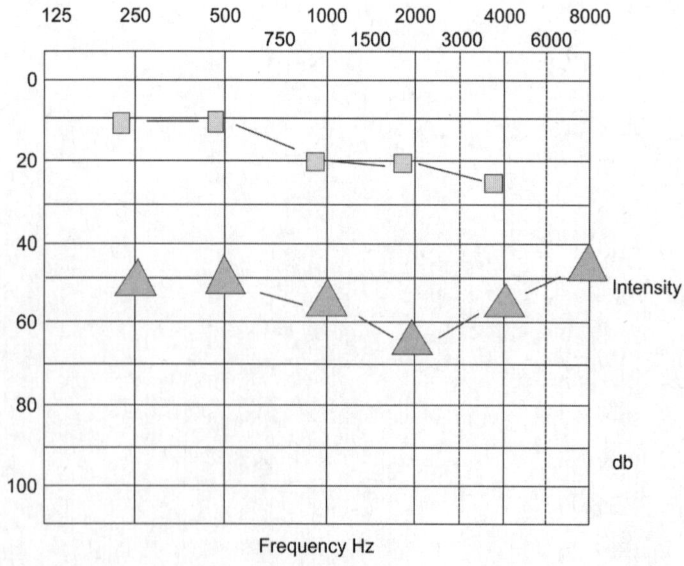

Otosclerosis

Other Options and Audiograms

Noise-induced hearing loss-acoustic dip (dip at 4000 Hz) in a SNHL curve

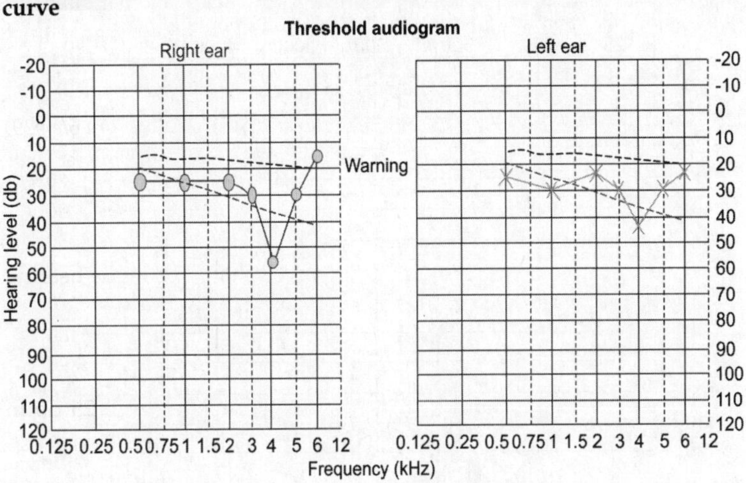

Meniere's Disease – It affects low frequency hearing loss in SNHL curve

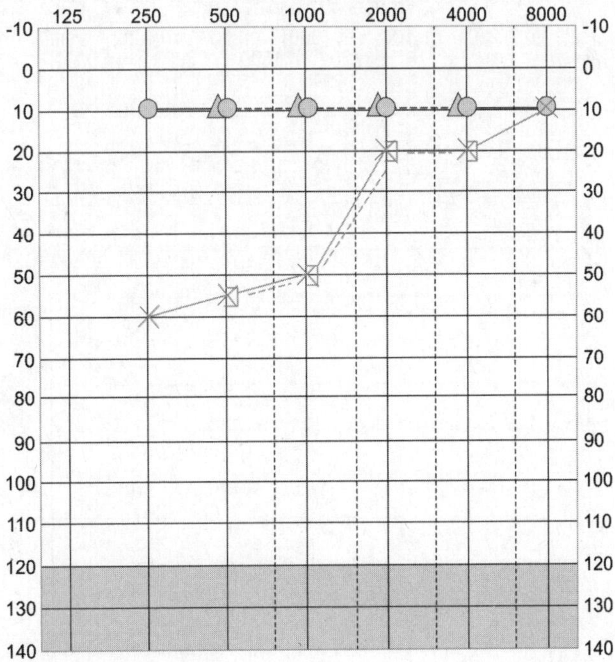

Presbycusis – affects high frequency hearing loss in SNHL curve

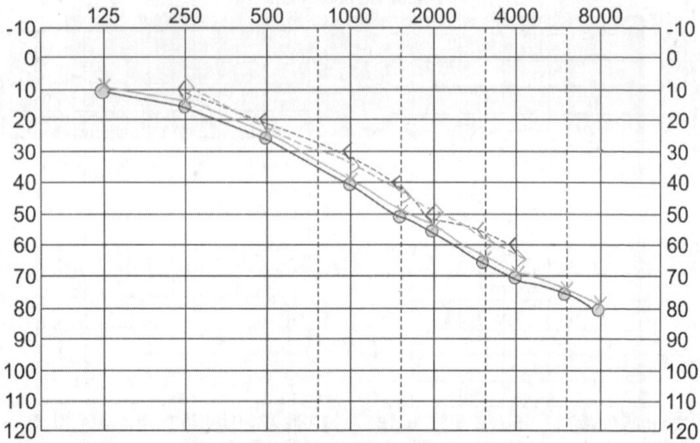

Ototoxicity – It affects higher frequencies in SNHL curve

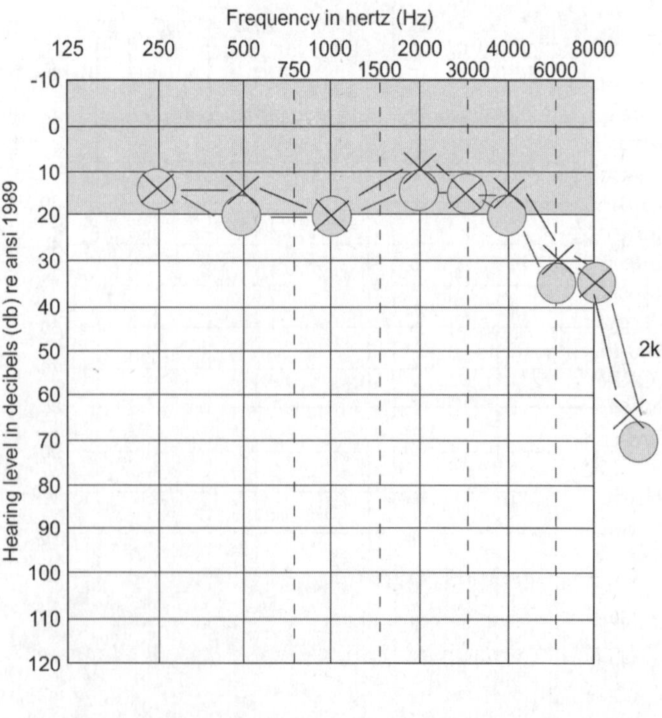

2. **Ans. d. Respiratory papillomatosis**

(Ref: Scott Brown 7/e – Volume 1, p1176)

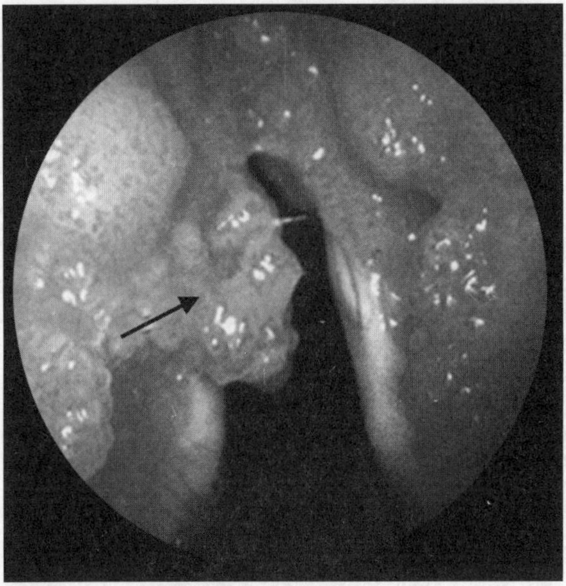

Juvenile onset recurrent respiratory papillomatosis (JORRP) is also known as laryngeal papilloma

- Caused by HPV subtypes 6 and 11, which are also responsible for causing anorectal condyloma
- Rare disease
- Infection can occur at birth (DIAGNOSED AT 2-4 YRS OF AGE)
- Most comman benign neoplasm of larynx in children
- Second most common cause of chronic childhood hoarseness
- 200-fold risk increases if mother has condyloma at delivery
- JORRP is more agrresive than adult variety
- Needs repeated surgical procedures to maintain the airway
- Presence of multiple grape-like warty lesions in larynx
  - Initial presentation is hoarseness and stridor
- If severe or size increases – recurrent respiratory infections and failure to thrive
- Treatment:
  - Intralesional cidofovir
  - Interferon therapy
  - HPV vaccine
  - Surgery (laser/cryosurgery)

Extra edge
- Laser-safe endotracheal tube (46%) and jet ventillation used for giving anesthesia
- CO_2/KTP lasers used
- PHOTODYNAMIC THERAPY used
- Indole-3-carbinol in diet improves symptoms

Croup and epiglottitis – are acute conditions, progressive increase of symptoms are not seen.
Vocal nodule has only hoarseness and doesn't give to airway obstruction

3. **Ans. a. Ohngren's line** *(Ref: Dhingra 6/e p207)*
A line from medial canthus of the eye to the angle of the mandible, used for maxillary cancer-staging.
- Anteroinferior/infrastructure has good prognosis
- Superoposterior/suprastructure has poor prognosis
- Early extension (eye, skull base, pterygoids, and infratemporal fossa). Growths situated above this plane ⇒ suprastructural (poorer prognosis)

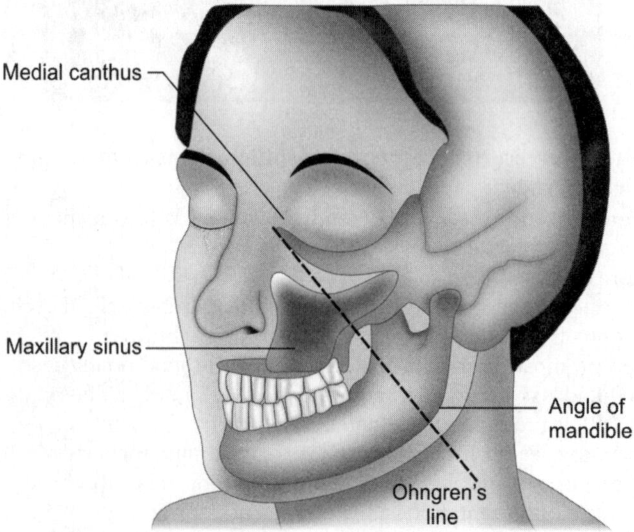

Anatomical landmark used in endolymphatic sac surgery is **Donaldson's line**.
- This is an imaginary line drawn posteriorly from the course of the horizontal semicircular canal.
- The line should course perpendicular to that of the posterior semicircular canal.

➢ The endolymphatic sac is located inferior to this line.

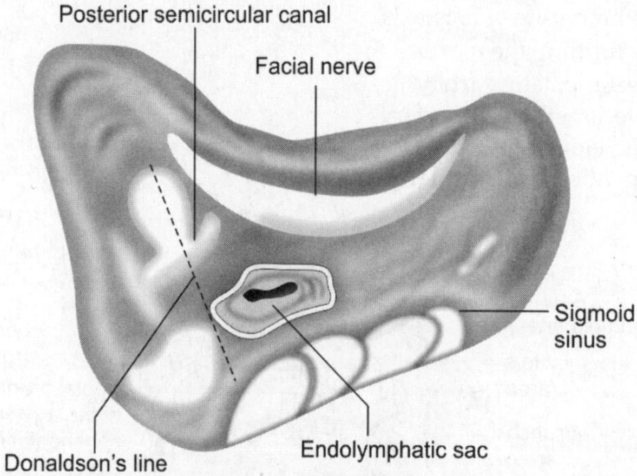

Frankfurt line: Skull is oriented so that the inferior margins of orbits and superior margins of EAC are horizontal. This is known as Frankfurt plane and the line joining them is known as Frankfurt line.

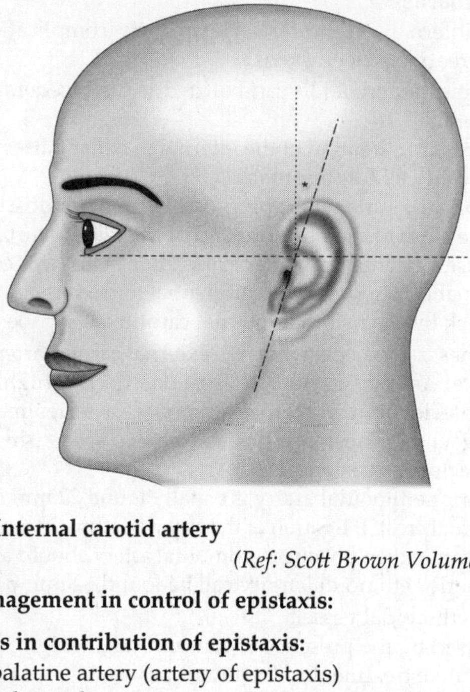

4. Ans. d. Internal carotid artery

(Ref: Scott Brown Volume 2, 7/e p1602)

Surgical management in control of epistaxis:

Major vessels in contribution of epistaxis:

➢ Sphenopalatine artery (artery of epistaxis)
➢ Ethmoidal vessels

Little area (Kiesselbach's plexus)

Most common site of epistaxis

Arteries forming the plexus:

- Greater palatine artery
- Anterior ethmoidal artery
- Sphenopalatine artery
- Superior labial artery (facial artery)

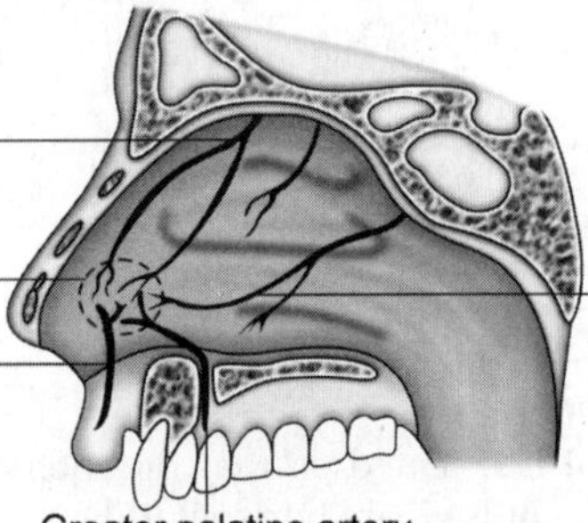

Surgical approaches:

Ligation of internal carotid artery has high complications and not advisable in treatment of epistaxis

- Endoscopic cauterization can be tried if the bleeders are localized and accessible.
- If not accessible, ligation of the internal maxillary artery can be done through caldwell Luc approach.
- Sphenopalatine artery clipping can be done endoscopically. It is accessible close to the posterior end of the middle turbinate.
- In rare cases, external carotid artery ligation at the neck can be resorted to. External carotid artery is differentiated from the internal carotid in the neck by the fact that internal carotid artery does not give rise to branches in the neck, while the external carotid artery does so.
- Ethmoidal artery ligation: If epistaxis occurs high in the nasal vault, anterior and posterior ethmoidal arteries may be ligated using ligaclips. These arteries can be accessed using an external ethmoidectomy incision.
- The anterior ethmoidal artery is usually found 22 mm from the anterior lacrimal crest. If ligation of the anterior ethmoidal artery does not stop bleeding, then posterior ethmoidal artery should also be ligated. The posterior ethmoidal artery can be found 12 mm posterior to the anterior ethmoidal vessel.

Epistaxis caused by the presence of tumors both, benign and malignant, calls for definitive treatment of the tumor per se.

PREVENTIVE AND SOCIAL MEDICINE

QUESTIONS

1. **A researcher said he has discovers a new drug which is effective in chronic hypertensives with a p value of < 0.10. Which of the following is true regarding the same?**
   a. The test is 90% reproducible
   b. 90% of test results could have occurred by chance
   c. Not more than 10% of the people benefitted by the drug could be due to chance
   d. 90% of patients will be benefitted by giving the drug
2. **A radiotherapist prescribes a new drug combination of chemotherapy and immunotherapy for metastatic melanoma. It prolongs the survival. Which of the following is true in this situation?**
   a. Incidence reduces and prevalence increases
   b. Incidence remains the same and prevalence increases
   c. Incidence reduces and prevalence remains the same
   d. Incidence increases and prevalence reduces
3. **A patient was sputum negative for TB, but chest X-ray was suggestive for TB. Which is the next step according to RNTCP?**
   a. Liquid culture b. CB-NAAT
   c. Line probe assay d. None of the above
4. **Below is the graph of CD4 count in HIV patients. From the graph below identify the mean CD4 count:**

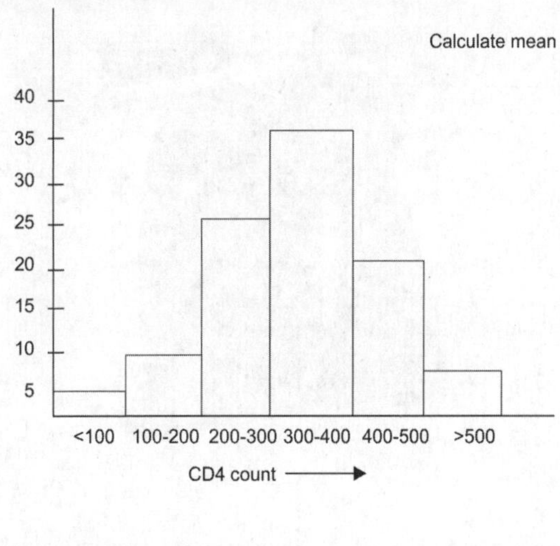

a. 350
b. Above 350
c. Below 350
d. Between 300-400

5. **Which point in the below natural history of disease marks the onset of symptoms?**

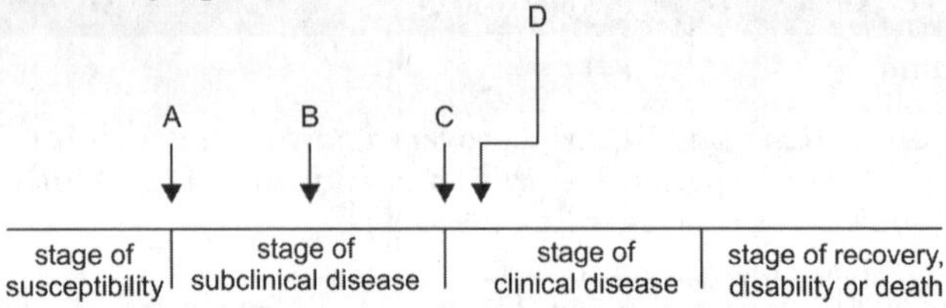

a. A
b. B
c. C
d. D

6. **A study was conducted with the objective to compare the incidence of postpartum depression in mother as compared to the sex of the child. For assessment Edinburg depression scaled score (EDSS) was used. The study was divided into mothers with male baby as one group to be compared with mothers with female baby. Which of the following statistical test will be used to determine the association?**

a. Students t-test
b. Chi-square test
c. ANOVA
d. Paired t-test

7. **Which of the following wastes are disposed in the bag shown below?**

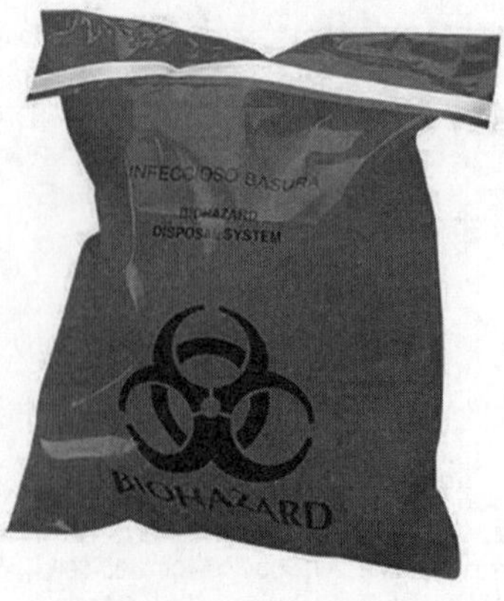

a. Anatomical waste
b. Sharp waste
c. Urine bags
d. Soiled waste

8. **A new test in red line has been designed to diagnose a disease condition. The test is being applied to both normal and diseased population. The graph of which is given below. Which of the following is correct regarding the test?**

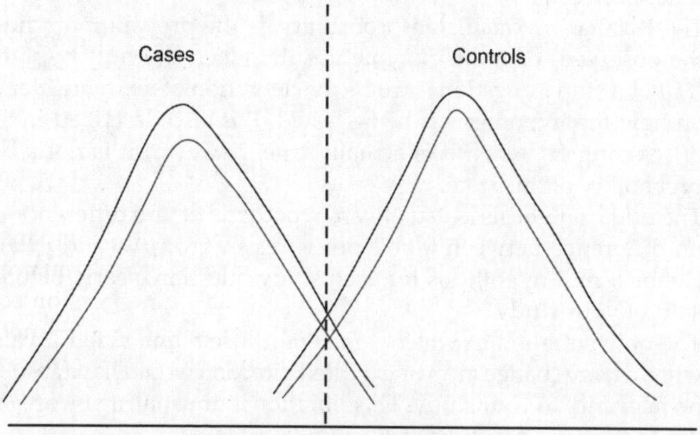

a. High sensitivity and high specificity
b. High sensitivity and low specificity
c. Low sensitivity and low specificity
d. Low sensitivity and high specificity

9. **The following are the disease frequencies in a population. Based on the number of cases which of the following is the correct match?**
Disease 1: Number of cases last week 42 this week 43
Disease 2: Number of cases last week 2 and present week 42
Disease 3: Number of cases last week 6 and present week 1

a. Endemic, epidemic, sporadic
b. Endemic, sporadic, epidemic
c. Sporadic, endemic, epidemic
d. Pandemic, endemic, sporadic

EXPLANATIONS

1. **Ans. c. Not more than 10% of the people benefitted by the drug could be due to chance**

(Ref: Oxford Handbook of Medical Statistics, p248)

P value is probability

- It lies between 0 to 1
- The P value, or calculated probability, is the probability of finding the observed, or more extreme, results when the **null hypothesis (H_0)** of a study question is true—the definition of 'extreme' depends on how the hypothesis is being tested. P is also described in terms of rejecting **H_0** when it is actually true, however, it is not a direct probability of this state.
- The null hypothesis is usually an hypothesis of "no difference", e.g. no difference between blood pressures in group A and group B. Define a null hypothesis for each study question clearly before the start of your study.
- The only situation in which you should use a **one sided** P value is when a large change in an unexpected direction would have absolutely no relevance to your study. This situation is unusual, if you are in any doubt then use a **two sided** P value.
- When presenting P values some groups find it helpful to use the asterisk rating system as well as quoting the P value:
  - $P < 0.05$ *
  - $P < 0.01$ **
  - $P < 0.001$
- Most authors refer to **statistically significant** as $P < 0.05$ and **statistically highly significant** as $P < 0.001$ (less than one in a thousand chance of being wrong).
- The asterisk system avoids the woolly term "significant"

Type I error:

- Is the incorrect rejection of the null hypothesis
- Maximum probability is set in advance as alpha
- Is not affected by sample size as it is set in advance
- Increases with the number of tests or end points (i.e. do 20 rejections of H_0 and 1 is likely to be wrongly significant for alpha = 0.05).

Type II error:

- Is the incorrect acceptance of the null hypothesis
- Probability is beta
- Beta depends upon sample size and alpha
- Can not be estimated except as a function of the true population effect

- Beta gets smaller as the sample size gets larger
- Beta gets smaller as the number of tests or end points increases.

2. **Ans. b. Incidence remains the same and prevalence increases**

(Ref: Park 24/e, p66)

- Incidence—New cases occurring
- Prevalence—Both new and old cases
- **Prevalence = Incidence × Duration**

Here the number of cases increase because the life span is prolonged. But there is no change in the incidence, since the treatment does not prevent melanoma, only treats it.

- Keep in mind that both I and P can change over time.

Prevalence increases when:

- Long- term survival rates increase (e.g. heart disease: better life-style, better drug compliance –> patient will live longer).

Prevalence decreases when:

- A new effective treatment is available.
- More rapid recovery from certain disease.
- More people dying from certain disease.

Both, prevalence and incidence decrease when:

- Preventive measures take place: vaccines, behavioral risk factors are reduced, reduced contacts between infected and noninfected people.

Incidence	Number of new cases occurring in a defined population during specified period of time usually expressed per 1000 population Incidence can be calculated from cohort study.
Prevalence	All the cases, current and old existing at a given point in time or over a period of time in a given population. It is determined by cross sectional study.
Point prevalence	Number of cases of the disease at a single point of time. The essential feature is that the study subjects are examined only once.
Period prevalence	A combination of the initial point prevalence and the subsequent incidence gives us the period prevalence. Period prevalence = (Initial point prevalence + Incidence)

3. **Ans. b. CB-NAAT**

(Ref: Technical and Operational Guidelines for TB Control in India, 2016)

- CB NAAT is Cartridge Based Nucleic Acid Amplification Test:
  - The gene expert TB test detects DNA sequences specific for M. Tuberculosis and Rifampicin resistance by PCR.
  - It is based on cepheid gene expert system, a platform for rapid and simple to use nuclei acid amplification tests (NAAT).
  - Results are obtained within 90 minutes.

Diagnostic algorithm for pulmonary TB New guideline

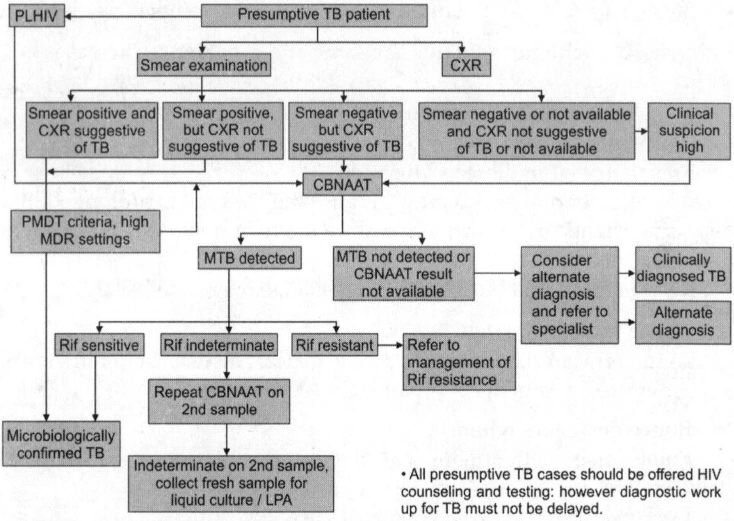

4. Ans. d. Between 300-400

(Ref: Oxford Handbook of Medical Statistics, p182)

Construct a table:

CD4 count	Number of people
< 100	5
100-200	10
200-300	25
300-400	35
400-500	20
> 500	5

CD4 count	Mid point	Number of people (n)	Mid point × N
0-100	50	5	250
100-200	150	10	1500
200-300	250	25	6250
300-400	350	35	12250
400-500	450	20	9000
500-1600	1050	5	5250
TOTAL		**100**	**34500**

- Mean = $x_1.n_1 + x_2.n_2 + \ldots\ldots$ = 34500/100 = 345
- So the best answer would be (d) between 300-400.

5. Ans. c. (C) *(Ref: Park 24/e, p40)*

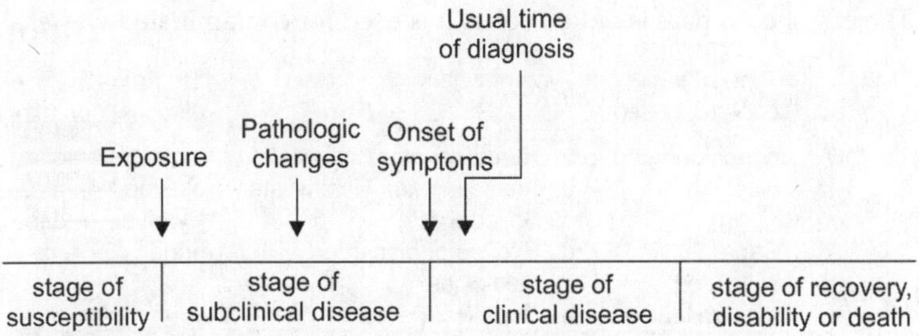

Source: The picture has been taken from CDC website.

- Point A marks the entry of infectious agent into the host
- Point B marks the subclinical phase where symptoms and signs are not visible, but the disease agent induces tissue and physiological changes
- Point C marks the clinical horizon when symptoms and signs appear
- Point D is present inside the clinical phase after the clinical horizon

Stage of subclinical disease, extending from the time of exposure to onset of disease symptoms, is usually called the **incubation period** for infectious diseases, and the **latency period** for chronic diseases.

6. Ans. b. Chi-square test *(Ref: Park 23/e, p852)*

- There are 2 groups
- Incidence is a qualitative variable—Presence of disease or Not
- The 2 groups are different.

Number of groups or condition	Parametric tests	Non parametric tests
Independent meas-ures, 2 groups	Unpaired t-test Or Student t-test	Chi-square test (large or small sample with Yate's correction) Fischer's test (small or large sample) Mann-Whitney U-test (Wilcoxon rank sum test)
Independent meas-ures, > 2 groups	ANOVA	Kruskal-Wallis test Chi-square test
Repeated measures, 2 conditions or Paired data	Paired t-test	Wilcoxon signed rank test, Mc-Nemar's test Chi-square test
Repeated measures, > 2 conditions	ANOVA	Friedman's test Chi-square test
Correlation test	Pearson	Spearman (Rho)
Regression	Simple linear or Nonlinear regression	Nonparametric regression

7. Ans. c. Urine bags *(Ref: Park 24/e p830)*

The bag shown here is of Red color. It is used for contaminated wastes.

Cat.	Type of bag/ container used	Type of waste	Treatment/ disposal options
Yellow	nonchlorinated plastic bags Separate collection system leading to effluent treatment system	a. Human anatomical waste b. Animal anatomyical waste c. Soiled waste d. Expired or discarded medicines e. Chemical waste f. Micro, Bio-technology and other clinical lab waste g. Chemical liquid waste	Incineration or plasma Pyrolysis or deep burial
Red	nonchlorinated plastic bags or containers	Contaminated waste (Recyclable) tubing, bottles, intravenous tubes and sets, catheters, urine bags, syringes (without needles) and gloves.	Auto/micro/hydro and then sent for recycling. Not be sent to landfill
White	(Translucent) Puncture, Leak, tamper proof containers	Waste sharps including metals	Auto or dry heat sterilizations followed by shredding or mutilation or encapsulation
Blue	Cardboard boxes with blue colored marking	Glassware	Disinfection or auto/micro/hydro and then sent for recycling.

8. Ans. b. High sensitivity and low specificity *(Ref: Park 23/e, p141)*

- The line in red shows the new test. The new test curve distribution is shorter than old thus, the 95% CI range of new test will be more precise than the old test.
- For a particular cut off point, sensitivity of new test will be high, since the 95% CI is precise for new test than old test. Now it's easy to answer the question. High sensitivity is achieved at the expense of decrease in specificity.

The definitions of sensitivity and specificity

- Sensitivity is simply a reflection of how many patients with the disease test positive.
- Specificity is a measure of your false positive rate.
- Note that sensitivity and specificity do not depend on disease prevalence

$$\text{Sensitivity} = \frac{TP}{TP + FN} = \frac{TP}{\text{Diseased}}$$

$$\text{Specificity} = \frac{TN}{TN + FP} = \frac{TN}{\text{Healthy}}$$

9. Ans. a. Endemic, epidemic, sporadic *(Ref: Park 24/e, p98)*

	Definitions of common terms
Epidemic	Occurrence of disease in excess of expected frequency
Pandemic	An epidemic affecting a large population over a large geographic area
Endemic	A disease occurring regularly in a population in expected frequency, without any importation from outside
Sporadic	Few, scattered cases of infection, which do not have any relation temporally/spatially. A disease occurring irregularly

MEDICINE

QUESTIONS

1. **On TFT analysis, TSH value was higher than normal and a subnormal free T4. Which of the following is the diagnosis?**
   a. Primary hypothyroidism
   b. Hyperthyroidism
   c. Subclinical hypothyroidism
   d. Secondary hypothyroidism

2. **A 20-year-old boy admitted to casualty with history of breathlessness following massage by mother. He had a history of hairline ankle fracture and was on a below knee cast which was removed recently. The most probable diagnosis is?**
   a. Pulmonary thromboembolism
   b. Pneumonitis
   c. Acute MI
   d. Septicemia

3. **All of the following is seen in CURB-65 *except*:**
   a. Respiratory rate of > 30/min
   b. Blood urea nitrogen value greater than 7 mmol/L
   c. Systolic blood pressure less than 100 mm Hg
   d. Confused state

4. **A middle aged woman with history of back pain came to OPD. On examination she was positive for Schober test. Her nose and ears were hyperpigmented. Your diagnosis is?**

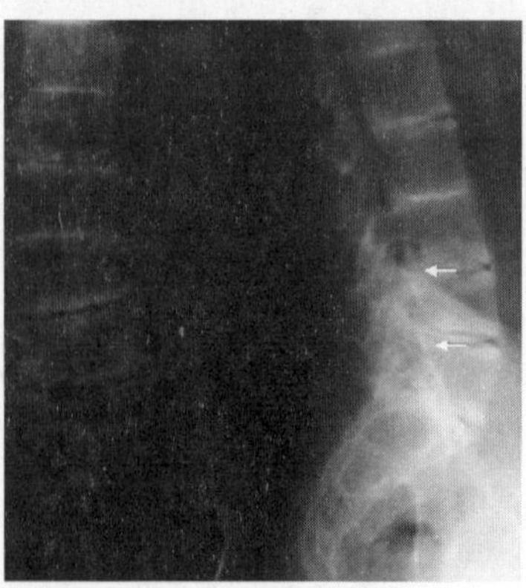

a. Hypoparathyroidism
b. Ochronosis
c. Fluorosis
d. Ankylosing spondylitis

5. Which of the following are feature of Zika Fever *except*:

a. Conjunctivitis
b. Fever with arthritis
c. Guillain-Barré syndrome
d. Petechial rash

6. A young girl with the diagnosis of APML was treated medically. She developed fever and tachypnea and chest X-ray shows infiltrates. Which is the drug she should be given next?

a. Doxorubicin
b. Methotrexate
c. Dexamethasone
d. Cytarabine

7. A middle aged man presented with frontal bossing and large tongue and he had spade shaped hands. Which of the following tests will you do for diagnosis?

a. Thyroid hormone assay
b. Serum prolactin
c. Insulin like growth factor
d. Serum testosterone

8. Which is the most appropriate treatment for the patient suffering from below condition:

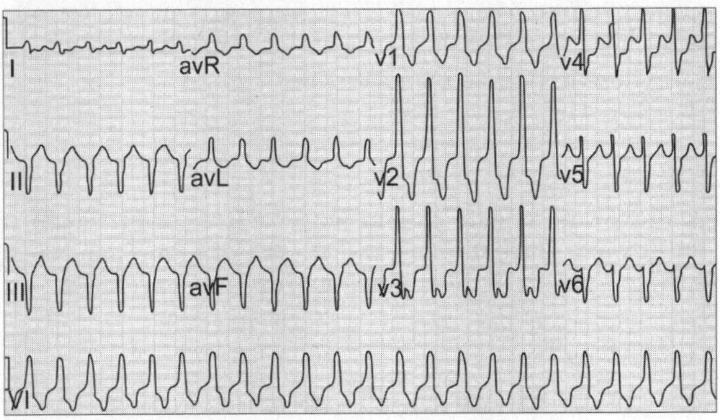

a. Lignocaine
b. DC cardioversion
c. Diazoxine
d. Lignocaine

9. **Definition of PUO includes all of the following *except*:**
   a. Fever persisting for more than 3 weeks
   b. Temperature more than 38.3 C
   c. Undiagnosed after one week of investigation
   d. Immuno-compromised status should be ruled out

10. **A 60-year-old man post MI had the following lab values LDL -127mg/dl, HDL -32 mg/dl, TGL-270 mg/dl. Which of the following must be his treatment plan?**
   a. Rosuvastatin + fenofibrate
   b. Atorvastatin 80 mg
   c. Rosuvastatin 20 mg
   d. Fenofibrate

11. **A 20-year-old female came with complaints of vomiting and decrease in movement of right leg. In the past she had episodes of violent and aggressive behaviour and abdominal pain. Which of the following is the most probable diagnosis?**
   a. Conversion disorder
   b. AIDP with migraine
   c. Right side paralysis
   d. Acute intermittent porphyria

12. **A 48-year-old smoker and hypertensive patient was on enalapril and hydrochlorothiazide. He had an episode of hemoptysis and was evaluated found to have bronchogenic carcinoma with brain metastasis. His lab values were Na -124 mg/dl, creatinine – 2.8 mg%, blood sugar 112 mg/dl, blood urea - 24 mg/dl, serum osmolality – 285/mosm, urine osmolality-350 msom, 24 hour urinary sodium 110 and BP 150/90 mmHg. Which of the following is the most probable diagnosis of the low sodium values?**
   a. Diuretic induced hyponatremia
   b. SIADH
   c. Cerebral salt wasting syndrome
   d. Pseudohyponatremia

13. **A 40-year-old female patient with NYHA class III heart failure with dyspnea, pedal edema and K levels of 4.5 mg% and creatinine 2.5 mg%. Which of the following drug is best avoided?**
   a. Spironolactone
   b. Carvedilol
   c. Enalapril
   d. Digoxin

14. **Which of the following is not a feature of Myasthenia Gravis?**
   a. Ptosis
   b. Normal pupillary reflux
   c. Muscle fatigue
   d. Absent reflex

15. **A patient presented with fracture of femur. On 3rd day of admission he developed sudden breathlessness. Which of the following is the most common cause?**
    a. Pulmonary hypertension b. Post-trauma MI
    c. Fat embolism d. Hypovolemic shock

16. **A patient came with complaints of high grade fever and altered sensorium. He was diagnosed to be suffering from meningococcal meningitis. Which of the following is the most appropriate empirical treatment option?**
    a. Ceftriaxone b. Cefotetan
    c. Penicillin G d. Cefoxitin

17. **A young male came with complaints of ascending weakness in lower limbs and upper body. There was no history of trauma. Which of the following is the next investigation?**
    a. Serum calcium b. Serum potassium
    c. Serum magnesium d. Serum sodium

18. **A lady delivered a normal vaginal delivery and was discharged. On third day she came back with fever, tachycardia and seizures. Fundus showed papilledema with no focal deficits. Diagnosis?**

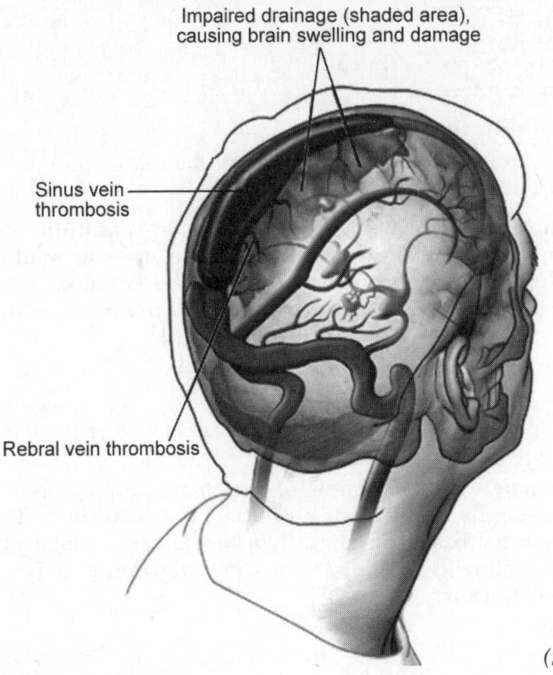

(See Color Plate 10)

a. Meningitis
b. Acute migraine
c. Cortical vein thrombosis
d. Subarachnoid haemorrhage

19. Which of the following features of stroke need not be treated:

a. Spasticity
b. Neglect
c. Dysphagia
d. Fever

20. A 40-year-old patient came with complaints of spikes of fever and difficulty in breathing. Transesophageal echo found out vegetations in the heart. The culture showed positive for Burkholderia cepaciae. Which of the following is the first line management?

a. Carbapenems and 3rd generation cephalosporins
b. Aminoglycosides and colistin
c. Cefepime and Tigecycline
d. Cotrimoxazonle with 3rd generation cephalosporin

21. Window period for thrombolysis in case of stroke is?

a. One and half hour
b. Two and half hour
c. Three and half hour
d. Four and half hour

22. (1–3)-β-D glucan assay can be used in all of the following infections *except*?

a. Invasive aspergillosis
b. Invasive candidiasis and candidemia
c. Pneumocystis jiroveci pneumonia
d. Invasive cryptococcosis

23. 'A' wave on JVP is for:

a. Atrial contraction
b. Ventricular relaxation
c. Ventricular filling
d. Atrial filling

24. A young male admitted with history of altered sensorium and hydrophobia. A suspicion of rabies was made and you want to diagnose the condition. You have taken corneal scrapings from the patient and which of the following tests will you do to confirm your diagnosis?

a. Seller stain for negri bodies
b. Indirect immunofluorescence
c. Real time PCR
d. Viral culture

25. A young female with complaints of bone pain and abdominal cramps. His family gives history of abnormal behaviour. The consultant doctor based on clinical feature made a diagnosis. Which of the following will be the best investigation to arrive at a definitive diagnosis?

a. Sestamibi scan
b. MRI
c. CT scan
d. Ultrasonogram

EXPLANATIONS

1. Ans. a. Primary hypothyroidism *(Ref: Harrison 19/e p2293)*

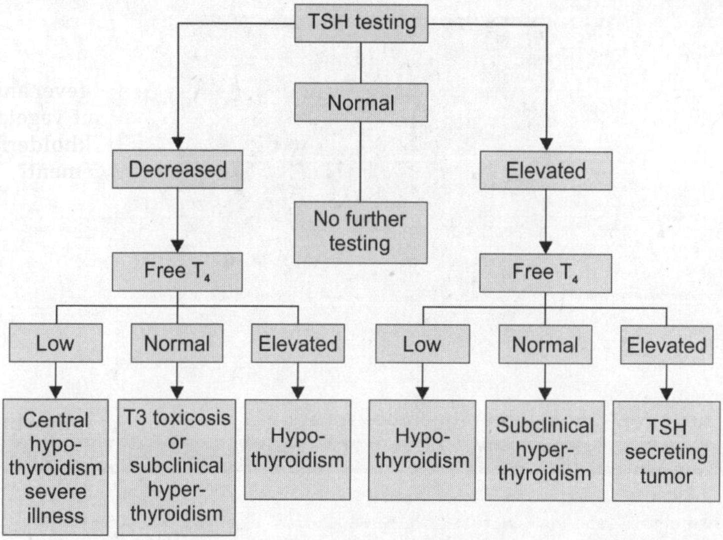

TSH is the most sensitive and the earliest indicator* of Thyroid function as the half-life of TSH is 1.5 to 3 hours.

Table showing the interpretation of Thyroid Function Tests and Pathology

Serum T3	Serum T4	Serum TSH	Inference
Normal	Normal	Normal	Euthyroid status
Elevated	Elevated	Decreased	Hyperthyroidism or toxicity
Normal	**Normal**	**Elevated**	**Subclinical hyperthyroidism**
Low	Low	Elevated	Hypothyroidism
Normal	**Normal**	**Elevated**	**Subclinical hypothyroidism**

Extra Edge
- Total T3 80-190 ng/dl
- Free T4 1.0-3.0 ng/dL
- Free T3 0.25-0.65 ng/dL

2. **Ans. a. Pulmonary thromboembolism** *(Ref: Harrison 19/e p1631)*

Boy was immobilised for long (fracture and below knee cast) it is a known risk factor for DVT (deep vein thrombosis) Upon massage the clot would had been dislodged causing pulmonary embolism leading to breathlessness and admission.

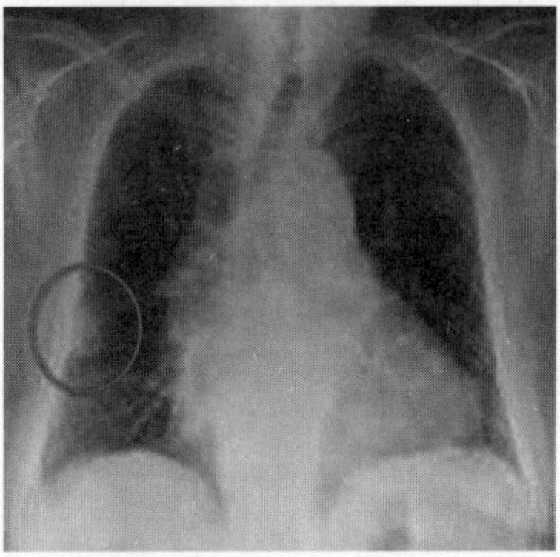

Causes for Venous Thromboembolism are

Stasis	Hypercoagulability	Endothelial Injury
❍ Hospitalization ❍ Immobilization ❍ Long air travel ❍ Spinal cord injury ❍ Advanced age ❍ Obesity	❍ Factor V Leiden ❍ Homocysteinemia ❍ Factor 7, 8, 9, 11 elevation ❍ Hyperfibrinogenemia ❍ Prothrombin gene mutation ❍ Antithrombin deficiency ❍ Protein C, S deficiency ❍ APLS ❍ Activated Protein C resistance ❍ Pregnancy ❍ Malignancy ❍ Nephrotic syndrome ❍ HRT and OCP use ❍ Puerperium	❍ Major surgery ❍ Varicose veins ❍ IV cannulation ❍ Trauma

- **Most common presentation of a DVT is pain and swelling** usually in the calf, on one side. But bilateral presentation is seen in 30% of individuals.
- **Homan's sign** – Dorsiflexion of the ankle causes pain in the calf
- **Moses sign** – Squeezing of the calf muscles causes pain in the calf
- Scores used to predict the risk of acquiring DVT include **Roger's score and Caprini score**.
- Criteria used to predict the risk of acquiring Pulmonary Embolism is **Modified Well's**

- **Investigation of choice for diagnosing PE is CT pulmonary angiography**
- Treatment includes Anticoagulation and observation, and in other cases catheter directed thrombolysis or embolectomy is being done. To prevent pulmonary embolism, **Inferior vena caval filters** are being used.

3. Ans. c. Systolic blood pressure less than 100 mm Hg

(Ref: CMBT 2017, p272)

There are two widely used clinical prediction rules available to guide admission and triage decisions in medicine emergencies.

- Pneumonia Severity Index (PSI)
- CURB-65.

Confusion
Urea >7mmol/l
Respiratory rate ≥30
Blood pressure: systolic <90mmHg or diastolic ≤60mmHg
Age ≥65 years
(Give score of 1 for each feature present)

CURB-65 score	Severity	Where to treat
0	Low	Home
1	Low	Home
2	Moderate	Hospital
3-5	High	Hospital: assess for ITU admission

Important:
Pneumonia severity scores (such as the CURB-65) must be used in conjunction with **clinical judgement** when assessing the severity of a pneumonia case

CURB-65 score is used to assess pneumonia severity. (especially for community acquired pneumonia)

CURB-65 is less discriminating at low mortality but excellent at identifying patients with high mortality who may benefit from ICU-level care.

4. Ans. b. Ochronosis *(Ref: Harrison 19/e p435.e-5)*

The problem is between ochronosis and AS.

The following is line from Harrison (Page.2172)

"Ochronosis can produce a phenotype that is clinically and radiographically similar to AS."

Now with another hint of hyperpigmented ear lobes, it is easy to narrow down to a Ochronosis (based on the clinical hint of pigmentation).

Schober test:

- Determines lumbar spine flexibility and motion and it is not specific for AS. It can be positive in any condition causing decreased lumbar spine motion.
- X-ray shows IV disc calcification which can occur in both AS and ochronosis

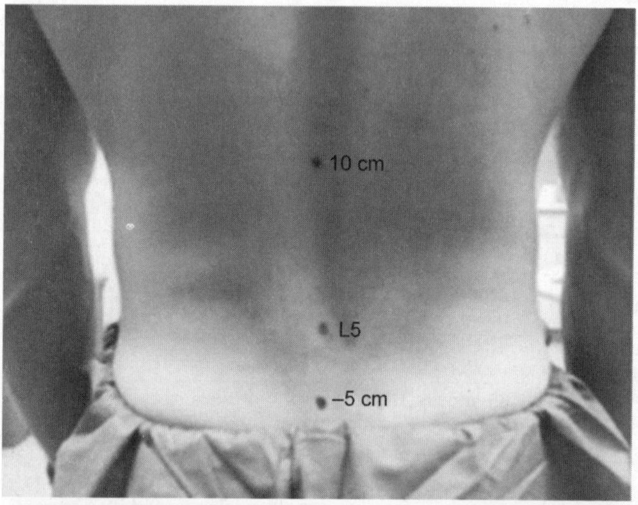

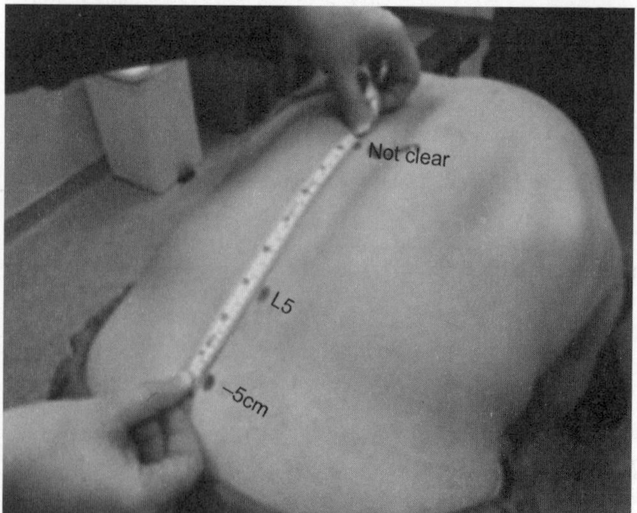

Ochronosis (Alkaptonuria)

Alkaptonuria is a rare (frequency 1:200,000) disorder of tyrosine catabolism in which deficiency of homogentisate 1,2-dioxygenase (also known as homogentisic acid oxidase) leads to excretion of large amounts of homogentisic acid in urine and accumulation of oxidized homogentisic acid pigment in connective tissues (ochronosis).

Triad:

- Homogentisic aciduria
- Pigmentation of cartilage
- Degenerative ochronic arthropathies usually in the fourth decade of life especially in spine, hip and knees.

"Ochronotic arthritis is heralded by pain, stiffness, and some limitation of motion of the hips, knees, and shoulders. Acute arthritis may resemble rheumatoid arthritis, but small joints are usually spared".

5. **Ans. d. Petechial rash** *(Ref: CDC and WHO)*

"Zika Fever was discussed in exclusive FB forum, 2 days before AIIMS exam.!"

Maculopapular rash and NOT petechial rash is a feature.

Symptoms of Zika virus
❍ Macular or Papular rash (90% of patients)
❍ Fever (65%)
❍ Arthritis or arthralgia (65%)
❍ Nonpurulent conjunctivitis (55%)
❍ Myalgia (48%),
❍ Headache (45%)
❍ Retro-orbital pain (39%)
❍ Edema(19%)
❍ Vomiting (10%)

Transmission:

Zika virus is primarily transmitted to people through the bite of an infected mosquito from the Aedes genus, mainly Aedes aegypti in tropical region.

Diagnosis:

- High index of suspicion
- Travel to epidemic or endemic areas
- Blood and body fluids for testing
  - ❑ Nucleic acid testing (NAT) testing (onset of symptoms < 7 days)
  - ❑ Serology (IgM detection) (onset of symptoms ≥ 7 days)

Treatment:

- Zika virus disease is usually mild and requires no specific treatment.
- People sick with Zika virus should get plenty of rest, drink enough fluids, and treat pain and fever with common medicines
- Pregnant women → kids develop microcephaly. Look out for EBOLA in coming exams

UNICEF Handout on EBOLA:

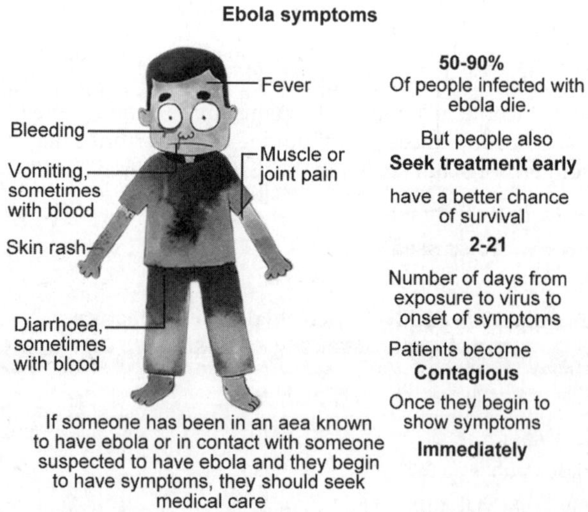

6. **Ans. c. Dexamethasone** *(Ref: Harrison 19/e p686)*

A well know side effect of ATRA (All-trans retinoic acid) **is differentiation syndrome:**

Differentiation syndrome – Clinical Features
❍ Fever
❍ Neutrophilia
❍ Hypoxia
❍ Pulmonary infiltrates
❍ Fluid overload

Pathogenesis:

- Tretinoin decreases the frequency of DIC but produces another complication called the APL differentiation syndrome within the first 3 weeks of treatment, it is characterized by fever, fluid retention, dyspnea, chest pain, pulmonary infiltrates, pleural and pericardial effusions, and hypoxemia

- The syndrome is related to adhesion of differentiated neoplastic cells to the pulmonary vasculature endothelium.

Treatment

- Glucocorticoids, chemotherapy, and/ or supportive measures can be effective for management of theAPL differentiation syndrome.
- Temporary discontinuation of tretinoin is necessary in cases of severe APL differentiation syndrome (i.e. patients developing renal failure or requiring admission to the intensive care unit due to respiratory distress).
- The mortality rate of this syndrome is about 10%.

7. **Ans. c. Insulin like growth factor** *(Ref: Harrison 19/e p2269)*

The patient has all clinical features of acromegaly.

Hot Acromegaly

- **H** eart failure/hypertension
- **O** edema
- **T** eeth spaced widely
- **A** ppearance/Amenorrhea
- **C** arpal tunnel syndrome/course skin/voice
- **R** eek
- **O** ily skin
- **M** yopathy
- **E** yes (prominent supra-orbital ridge)
- **G** oiter/gain weight/galactorhea
- **A** rthropathy
- **L** arge tongue and nose
- **Y** onset early

Etiology:

Excess Growth Hormone Secretion	Prevalence %
Pituitary	98
Densely or sparsely granulated GH cell adenoma	60
Mixed GH cell and PRL cell adenoma	25
Mammosomatotrope cell adenoma	10
Plurihormonal adenoma	
GH cell carcinoma or metastases	
Multiple endocrine neoplasia 1 (GH cell adenoma)	
McCune-Albright syndrome	
Ectopic sphenoid or parapharyngeal sinus pituitary adenoma	
Extrapituitary tumor	
Pancreatic islet cell tumor	< 1
Lymphoma	

Contd...

Contd...

Excess Growth Hormone–Releasing Hormone Secretion	
Central	< 1
Hypothalamic hamartoma, choristoma, ganglioneuroma	< 1
Peripheral	< 1
Bronchial carcinoid, pancreatic islet cell tumor, small cell lung cancer, adrenal adenoma, medullary thyroid carcinoma, pheochromocytoma	

Investigation:

- Screening IOC – IGF-1
- Confirmatory and gold standard – OGTT

Treatment:

- TOC – Surgery
- If failed/Surgery cannot be done – Octreotide/Pasireotide or Pegvisomant (GH receptor antagonist)

Familial Acromegaly:

- Familial acromegaly is a rare disorder in which family members may manifest either acromegaly or gigantism.
- A subset of families with a predisposition for familial pituitary tumors, especially acromegaly, have been found to **harbor germline mutations in the AIP gene**, which encodes the aryl hydrocarbon receptor interacting protein

High Yield (Endocrinology)

	Test	Comments
Acromegaly	Serum IGF-I Oral glucose tolerance test with GH obtained at 0, 30, and 60 min	Interpret IGF–I relative to age and sex-matched controls Normal subjects should suppress growth hormone to <1 g/L
Prolactinoma	Serum PRL	Exclude medications MRI of the sella should be ordered if PRL is elevated
Cushing's disease	24–h urinary free cortisol Dexamethasone (1 mg) at 11 p.m. and fasting plasma cortisol measured at 8 A.M. ACTH assay	Ensure urine collection is total and accurate Normal subjects suppress to < 5 g/dL Distinguishes adrenal adenoma (ACTH suppressed) from ectopic ACTH or Cushing's disease (ACTH normal or elevated)

Acromegaly: (Pic Harrison)

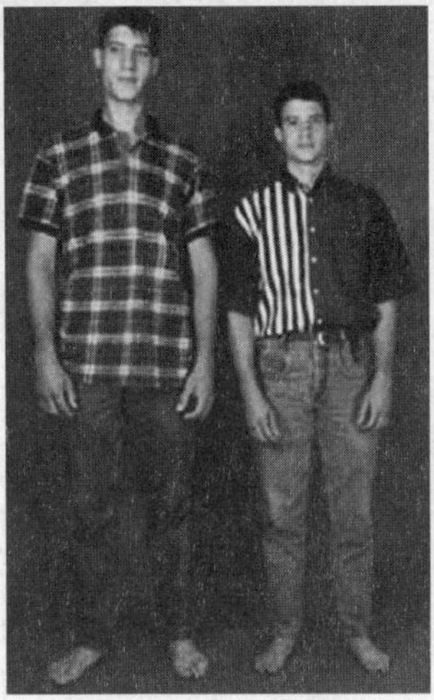

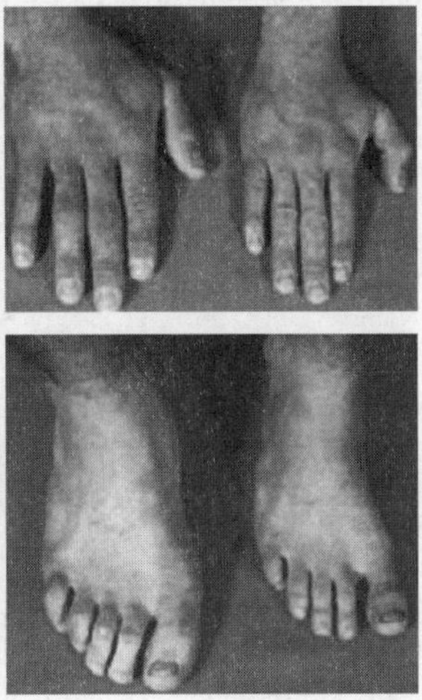

8. **Ans. b. DC cardioversion**

This is a broad complex regular tachycardia. Any broad complex regular tachycardia should be taken as VT unless proved otherwise.

Here there is no history suggestive of hemodynamic stability given in the question.

Treatment options include

- Amiodarone for stable patients
- DCC for unstable patients (Higher success rate compare to drugs)

Taking into account the higher success rate and other options not a viable as a better treatment option, the best option here would be DC cardioversion.

Defibrillation	Cardioversion
Not synchronised	Synchronised on the R wave
For cardiac arrest	For periarrest tachyarrhythmias (unstable)
Higher energy joules	Lower energy joules
No escalating energy for next shock	Escalate for next shock (100-200-300-360J)

9. **Ans. c. Undiagnosed after one week of investigation**

(Ref: API Textbook of Medicine. Chapter 52)

- The question is based on the latest criteria for FUO.
- Differences with old and latest criteria for FUO.

Old (Petersdorf et al 1961)	Latest (Miller et al)
Fever > 38.3 C (101F) * 2 occasions	Fever > 38.3 C (101F) * 2 occasions
Duration > 3 weeks	Duration > 3 weeks
Diagnosis not certain after 1 week of IP evaluation	***REMOVED***
	No immunocompromised state
	Diagnosis not certain after history/exam and routine + obligatory investigations

Types of PUO

Category	Classic PUO	Nosocomial PUO	Neutropenic PUO	HIV PUO
Definition	> 3 wks or > 2 OPD visits or > 3 days of indoor investigation	> 3 days, not present or incubation on admission	> 3 days, absolute neutropenia (< 500/mL)	3 wks of outpatients or 3 days indoor
Leading causes	Infections, collagen vascular disorders, Cancers	LRTI (Lower respiratory tract infection), UTI, catheter sepsis, post operative complications	Infections but can be found in only 50%	Typical or atypical mycobacteria, CMV (cytomegalo virus). toxoplasma
Time course of disease	Months	Weeks	Days	Weeks to months
Tempo of investigations	Weeks	Days	Hours	Days to weeks

Work up protocol:

USG abdomen + neck (for lymph nodes)
If young – serology for collagen vascular disease

↓

CT chest (even if multiple CXR normal)

↓

CT abdomen and pelvis (even if USG normal)

↓

Bone marrow examination, CSF examination
(even nothing to suspect meningitis)
Scalene lymph node biopsy (even if not enlarged)

↓

Liver biopsy (even if no reason to suspect hepatic pathology)
(SOS biopsy of lesion shown in any radiological investigation can be done)

10. Ans. b. Atorvastatin 80 mg *(Ref: ACC/AHA Guidelines)*

Category 1:

- Use statins irrespective of cholesterol levels in ASCVD (MI/CAD/Angina/Stroke/TIA/PVD)

Category 2 :

- Based on Cholesterol levels in patients without ASCVD
  - LDL > 190 – High intensity statins (Moderate intensity if Age > 75)
  - LDL > 70 + DM + Age > 40 yrs
  - LDL > 70 + Age > 40 yrs
  - 10 yr CV risk > 7.5%

Note:

- Category 1- For all patients with clinical ASCVD – High intensity statins
- Category 2
  - For 'a'– High intensity
  - b/c/d alone – Moderate intensity statins
  - B or c + d – High intensity statins

Categories:

- If Age > 75 or intolerant to high intensity statins – Use Moderate intensity statins.
- High intensity statins – Atorvas 40 – 80 mg / Rosuvas 20-40 mg (Best with Atorvas 80 mg and Rosuvas 40 mg). Atorvas 20-40 mg and Rosuvas 5-10 mg is a moderate intensity statin.
- Fenofibrate not advocated unless TG > 500. Can be administered along with a moderate intensity statin. (No more adding fibrate to a statin is contraindicated). This is not a high quality data anyway.

With previous history of MI this patient will come under High intensity statin support.

11. Ans. d. Acute intermittent porphyria *(Ref: Harrison 19/e p2526)*

Above is classical definition of clinical symptoms in Acute Intermittent porphyria.

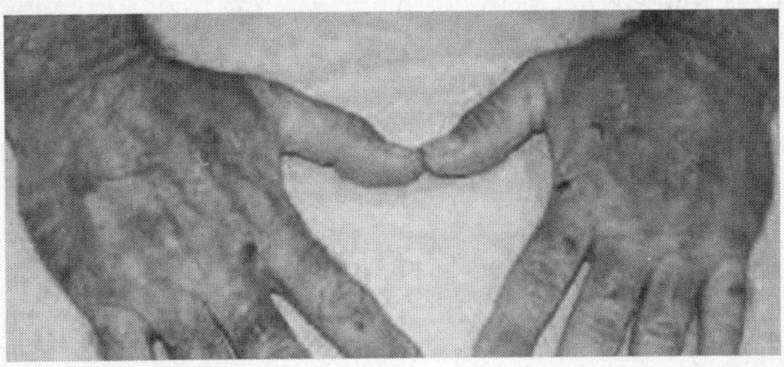

Acute Intermittent Porphyria:

- Most are asymptomatic
- AIP manifests after puberty, especially in women (due to hormonal influences)
- Symptoms are discrete
- Classic exam scenario:
  a. Young female
  b. Recurrent abdominal pain +/- vomiting
  c. Neuropsychiatric manifestations
  d. Concurrent hyponatremia – due to SIADH

Remember: Most common Porphyria is Porphyria cutanea tarda which has dermatologic manifestations.

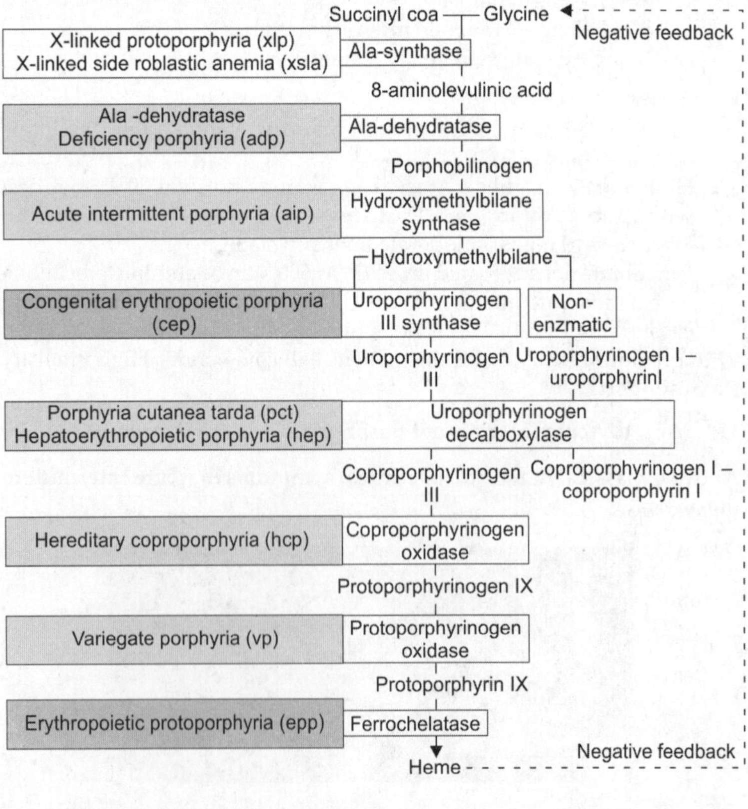

12. Ans. b. SIADH *(Ref: CMBT 2017, p885)*

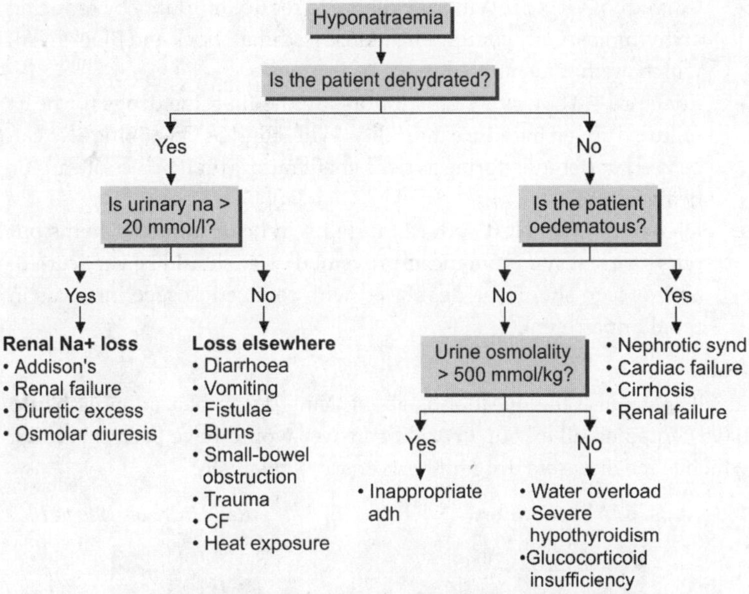

Presence of Bronchogenic cancer with brain metastasis present with paraneoplastic syndromes of which SIADH is most common.

Further lets try to rule out other options

Other options:

- Reduced Serum osmolality is not seen in Pseudohyponatremia as patients have normal osmolality
- Cerebral salt wasting syndrome patients are hypovolemic due to volume depletion hence these patients have hypotension.
- Diuretic induced hyponatremia will have urinary Na > 20 mmol/L and ECF volume will be decreased. Plus blood pressure owing to use of diuretics has to be low.

13. Ans. a. Spironolactone *(Ref: AHA guidelines)*

Spironolactone:

Contraindications for use of drug are –
❍ Serum creatinine = 2.5 mg/dL (men) and Serum creatinine = 2.0 (women)
❍ Low GFR
❍ Hyperkalemia

Other options

- Carvedilol – it is proved drug known to reduce mortality by reducing arrhythmias. Only contraindication is Asthma, shock and Blocks (AV) which are not mentioned in the qs.
- Enalapril – They as ACE inhibitors are the first line drugs for heart failure. Proven to reduce mortality. With High Sr Creatinine also can be used under monitoring as risk benefit ratio is high in case of chronic heart failure.
- Digoxin – Does NOT reduce mortality in heart failure patients but offers a great symptomatic improvement. Use should be very careful and dosage should be degreased with reduced dosage intervals in renal impairment.

Note:

Ideally – in case the question is about acute decompensation it should have contained all except – For that answer would have been carvedilol which is the only safe drug in this scenario – relatively.

14. Ans. d. Absent reflex *(Ref: Harrison 19/e p2703)*

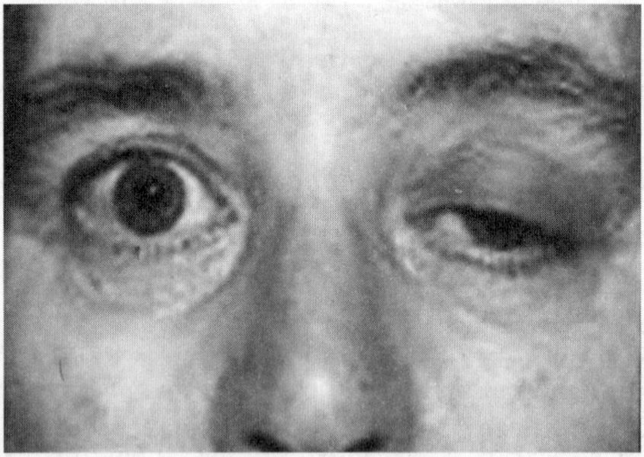

Myasthenia Gravis (MG) has normal DTR's, never lost

Myasthenia gravis:

- Progressive weakness caused by an autoantibody to the acetylcholine receptor on the neuromuscular endplate
  - Type II hypersensitivity reaction
  - Eventual destruction of the receptor
- Antibody synthesized in the thymus and removal of the thymus can lead to symptomatic improvement
- Occurs primarily in women 20–30 years, also can occur in men 70–80 years.

Evaluation

- Serology
  - Acetylcholine receptor (AChR) antibodies
  - Muscle-specific tyrosine kinase (MuSK) antibodies
- Edrophonium test ("Tensilon test")
  - Cholinesterase inhibitor which allows more ACh to present at the synapse
  - Positive test is the resolution of weakness with a regain of strength
  - Not used often
- Ice-pack test
  - Helpful in diagnosing myasthenia gravis in patients with prominent ptosis
  - Decreasing temperatures decrease acetylcholinesterase activity which results in increased ACh in the synaptic cleft.

15. Ans. c. Fat embolism *(Ref: Harrison 19/e p40-e4, 368)*

Reasons:

- Fat embolism syndrome occurs 24–72 hours after long bone Breathlessness is the earliest symptom.
- PE– usually beyond 4–5 days. Also the etiology usually finds mentions of prolonged and a history of surgery is usually there.

Extra Edge

Gurd and Wilson criteria used for diagnosis

- Major Criteria
  - Respiratory insufficiency
  - Cerebral involvement
  - Petechial rash
- Minor Criteria
  - Tachycardia
  - Fever
  - Jaundice
  - Retinal changes
  - Renal changes
- Laboratory Features
  - Microglobulinemia (required)
  - Thrombocytopenia
  - Elevated ESR
  - Anemia

One major and 4 minor criteria, plus fat microglobulinemia, must be present to formally diagnose fat embolism syndrome.

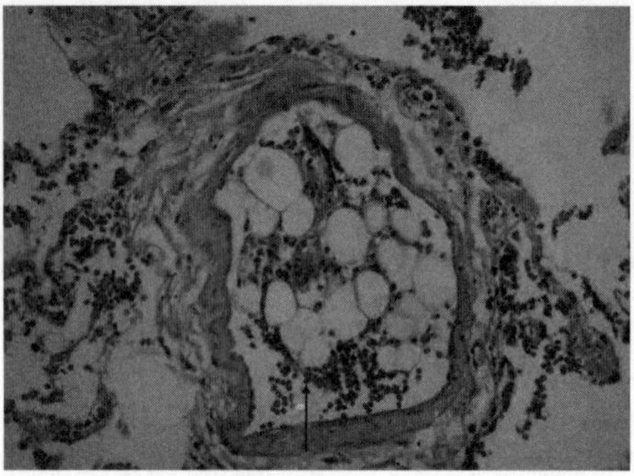

Fat Embolism Syndrome:

- Fat embolism is defined by the presence of fat globules in the pulmonary circulation.
- Fat embolism syndrome (FES) is a rare clinical syndrome that is most commonly associated with long bone (especially femur) and pelvic fractures
- The classic triad of findings includes:
    - Hypoxemia
    - Neurologic abnormalities, and
    - A petechial rash.
- Breathlessness is the earliest manifestation.
- Prevention is by **early immobilization**
- Treatment is generally supportive and steroids can be used in severe cases

16. Ans. a. Ceftriaxone *(Ref: Harrison 19/e p885)*

Empirical Regimen of Choice.

- Eventhough Penicillin is the DOC for SUSCEPTIBLE strains – penicillinase producing meningococcus is increasing and one cannot risk starting penicillin unless and until culture results are available.
- 3rd generation cephalosporins like cefotaxime/ceftriaxone are the empirical treatment of choice until culture reports are available.
- Once cultures show susceptibility of Meningococcus to penicillin – ceftriaxone/cefotaxime can be discontinued and penicillin can be started.

17. Ans. b. Serum potassium

- Hypokalemia (as well as hyperkalemia for that matters) can well produce ascending weakness very similar to GBS.
- So it is always imperative to check S. Potassium values in any suspected GBS case before proceeding to the diagnostic investigations and treatment.

Electrolyte imbalance and muscle disorders

- Sodium problems would not cause Muscular weakness.
- Hypocalcemia and Hypomagnesemia would have caused Tetany in the patient.
- Hypercalcemia would have other features apart from weakness

Extra Edge (GBS)

Differential diagnosis of GBS

- Myasthenia gravis
- Als
- Infectious myelitis (polio, west nile, other enteroviruses),
- Paralytic porphyria,
- Heavy metal poisoning,
- Toxin ingestion (botulism, ciguatoxin, tetrodotoxin),
- Tick paralysis,
- Multiple sclerosis,
- Carcinomatous meningitis

18. Ans. c. Cortical vein thrombosis *(Ref: Harrison 19/e p910)*

There can be three possible clinical scenarios/ diagnosis, which should be kept in mind while examining a female postpartum patient with headache and seizures.

- Eclampsia - no history favoring it
- CVT
- Pituitary hemorrhage / Sheehan's syndrome

Other Options

- Meningitis—without neck rigidity and a papilledema is rare (not possible, ruled out)
- Migraine – will not have seizures

Cortical vein thrombosis:

- The major risk factors for CVT in adults are prothrombotic conditions, oral contraceptives, pregnancy, malignancy, infection and head injury.
- The onset can be acute, subacute, or chronic.
- Headache (of gradual, acute, or thunderclap onset) is the most frequent symptom – Most common presentation
- They may be with or without vomiting, papilledema, and visual problems.. They may occur WITHOUT Focal Neurological deficits.
- Parenchymal brain lesions, including brain swelling, edema, venous infarction, or hemorrhagic venous infarction, may occur secondary to venous occlusion.
- **Brain MRI in combination with magnetic resonance (MR) venography** is the **most sensitive** examination technique for demonstrating the thrombus and the occluded Dural sinus or vein.

19. Ans. a. Spasticity *(Ref: Textbook of Stroke Medicine, p297)*

- Fever: Is deleterious in stroke patients. So it has to be treated.
- Spasticity: Overzealous Treatment affects the normal ambulation of patients. Hence treating spasticity as a rule is not always preferred, treating it is a double edged sword. It is specifically mentioned in books that Spasticity as a consequence of a stroke might in many cases also have a certain beneficiary compensatory aspect.
- Dysphagia: Dysphagia is serious and it poses a significant risk for aspiration and hence it has to be treated. Dysphagia in stroke is predominantly oropharyngeal type.
- Neglect is an inability to attend to, orient or explore the hemisphere contralateral to a brain lesion. Since right is dominant for selective attention, this syndrome is usually seen in right hemi stroke (36-80% patients) and affects awareness of left side. It has negative impact on daily activities and on functional recovery, hence it should be treated.

Neuroprotective agents:

Prolongation of tolerance of brain to ischemic long enough to allow other measures to be employed to mitigate ischemia. Agents used are:

- Hypothermia

20. Ans. d. Cotrimoxazonle with 3rd generation cephalosporin

(Ref: Harrison 19/e p1048, 1697)

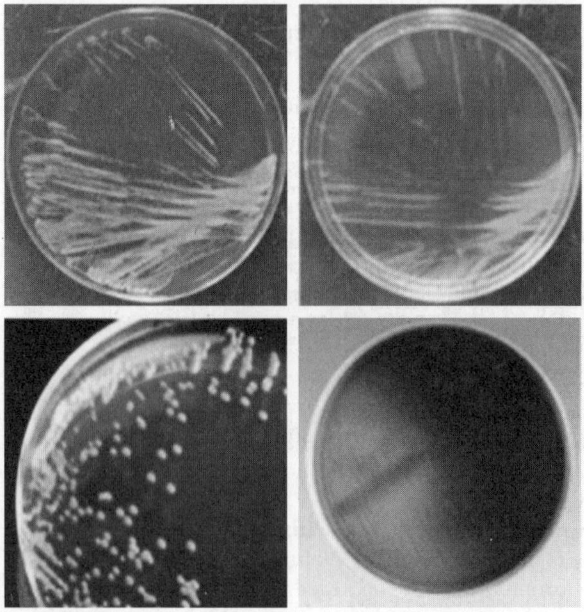

- Burkholderia cepacia is a chronic colonizer pathogen usually causing infection to immunocompromised or hospitalized patients.
- It is also associated with infections in patients with underlying lung disease, such as cystic fibrosis and chronic granulomatous disease.
- Management of these cases is difficult due to intrinsic resistance to most of the antibiotics including polymixins and aminoglycosides.

Effective agents for Burkholderia capecia
- Cotrimaxazole (40-45% sensitivity)
- Minocycline (38%)
- Meropenem > other carbapenems (26%)
- Ceftazidime (23%)
- Anti- pseudomonal penicillins/cephalosporins/quinolones
- Doxycycline. But minocycline is superior

Cotrimoxazole is the drug of choice for the treatment of infections caused by *B. cepacia* along with ceftazidime and meropenem, alone or in combination with other antibiotics.

It is innately resistant to various antimicrobial agents including polymyxins, aminoglycosides, chloramphenicol and b-lactams. Mechanisms conferring resistance include efflux pumps, production of b-lactamases and other modifying enzymes, as well as modification of antibiotic targets.

Note:
- In case of Cystic Fibrosis—Meropenem + cipro + Tobramycin nebulisation

21. Ans. d. Four and half hour *(Ref: Thrombolysis in Stroke guidelines)*

Window period for thrombolysis as per the current guideline is 4.5 hours.

C/I FOR THROMBOLYSIS
BP > 185/110 mm Hg
Plt < 1L/mm^3
Glucose < 50 or > 400 mg/dl
Heparin use in the last 48h
Rapidly improving symptoms
Elevated PT/aPTT/INR
Prior intracranial hemorrhage
Prior ischemic stroke within 3 months
Head injury in last 3 weeks
Major surgery in last 2 weeks
GI bleeding in the last 3 weeks

Contd...

Contd...

Coma/stupor
Recent MI
Consent could not be obtained
Age < 18 years
Pregnancy (relative – not absolute)
Onset of symptoms > 4.5h or timing unknown
CT scan showing bleeding / Edema of > 1/3rd of MCA territory

22. Ans. d. Invasive cryptococcosis *(Ref: CMBT 2017, p1291, 1336)*

1, 3 BD Glucan assay is utilized for the diagnosis of invasive aspergillosis, candidemia and PCP.

Accuracy of diagnostic testing for invasive fungal infections in the ICU				
Technique	**Sensitivity**	**Specificity**	**Advantages**	**Disadvantages**
Culture Methods	50%	100%	Gold standard; allows susceptibilities	Delay in diagnosis; low sensitivity
PCR Methods	90%	100%	Highest accuracy	Low commercial availability
β–D-glucan	70–100%	87–96%	Panfungal marker; high sensitivity and specificity	Many false–positive results; methodological concerns
Galactoman-nan	80–90%	80–90%	Increased accuracy for detection of Aspergillus in hematologic illnesses	Only for Aspergillus; many false–positive results; not useful in non-hematologic illnesses
Mannan or Antimannan Combination	60–89% 87%	80–84% 84%	God specificity and sensitivity with combined use	Results vary; limited experience

Measurement of biologic markers, such as the galactomannan Aspergillus antigen and the fungal wall component (1–3)-β-D-glucan, offers a noninvasive method for the detection of invasive fungal infections.

23. **Ans. a. Atrial contraction**

a' wave – Atrial contraction
'c' wave – Isovolumetric centricular contraction – causing bulging of Tricuspid valve into RA
'v' wave – atrial filling (venous filling)
'x' descent – atrial relaxation
' x' ' descent – pulling of atrial floor downward by active ventricular contraction
'y' descent – ventricular filling during diastole

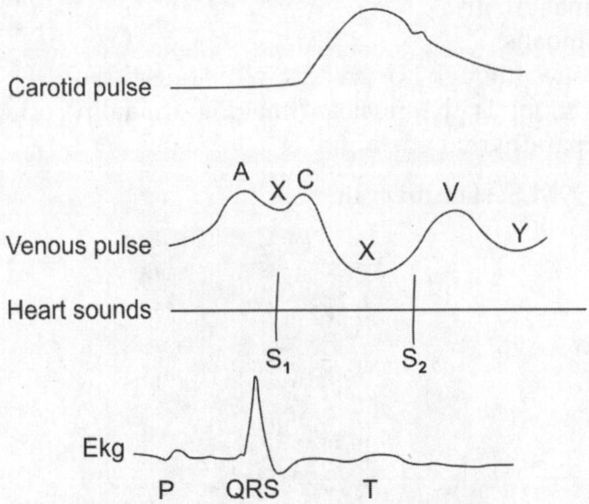

24. **Ans. d. Viral culture** *(Ref: Manson's Tropical Diseases 23/e p201)*

This is a repeat from AIIMS Nov 2016. The location of sample determines the test to be done.

The key points in the ante-mortem lab diagnosis of rabies encephalitis are:

- First of all Corneal impressions/scrapings are currently NOT preferred
- Negri bodies can be demonstrated only in the brain (Hippocampus -pyramidal fibers of Ammon's horn > Cerebellar purkinje fibres/ cortical neurons) and not found In skin, cornea, saliva or CSF samples.
- Viremia is not seen in rabies and hence BLOOD is NOT used for diagnosis.
    - Current antemortem diagnostic test of choice for rabies – DFA (Direct Fluorescent Antibody) in a skin sample obtained from the nape of the neck.
    - Samples used for DFA – Brain is the overall best tissue (especially postmortem). Skin samples are the best for antemortem diagnosis as there are risks involved in obtaining brain samples.

- Virus isolation through culture – Best specimens: Brain and Saliva. CSF, corneal smears and centrifuged urine can also be used.

No single test according to CDC/WHO is confirmatory. Multiple tests done in tandem/simultaneously are the best.

DFA followed by Virus isolation/Culture is confirmatory.

25. Ans. a. Sestamibi scan *(Ref: Harrison 19/e p2473)*

Clinical features are highly suggestive of (Primary) hyperparathyroidism.

This patient has some of the classic features described in the literature:

- Abdominal groans
- Psychic moans
- Renal stones (though not present in the question)

Tc 99m Sestamibi is the nuclear imaging modality utilized for the diagnosis of parathyroid adenoma.

Image of Tc 99M Sestamibi scan:

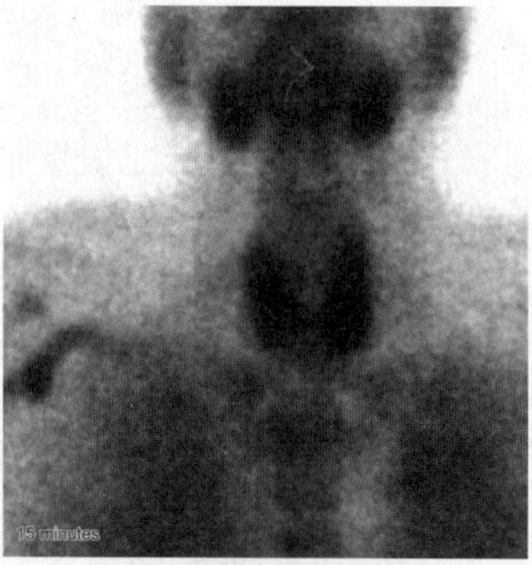

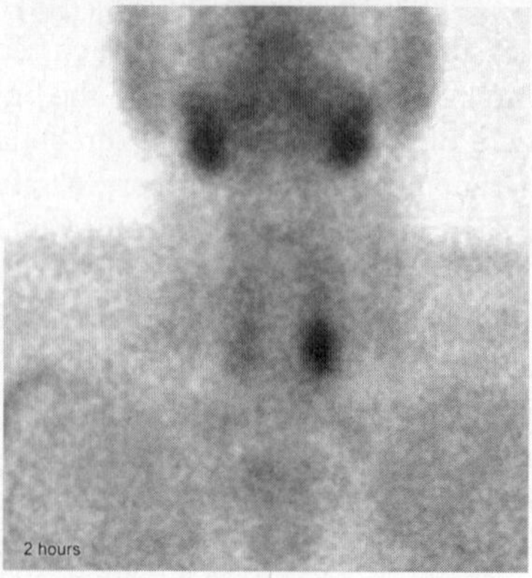

SURGERY

QUESTIONS

1. **A patient underwent a laparoscopic cholecystectomy and discharged on Day 1 after drain removal. On 3rd POD, the patient was febrile and came back for follow-up. On USG collection of 5 × 5 cm in the subhepatic space was observed. Next best step is:**
   a. Pigtail insertion and drainage
   b. Re-explore the wound and T tube insertion
   c. Give oral antibiotics and send patient home
   d. ERCP
2. **Primary survey in a traumatized patient all are true *except*:**
   a. Cervical X-ray is not mandatory
   b. Chest X-ray and pelvic X-ray are taken as a part of primary survey
   c. Hemodynamically unstable patient should not be sent for CT scan
   d. All patients should have chest X-ray – PA view only
3. **A mid-thirty female underwent surgery for breast cancer of 1.2 × 1 cm with positive axillary nodes. She completed radiotherapy and chemotherapy and now on tamoxifen. How will you follow-up the patient?**
   a. Yearly bone scans
   b. Routine physical examination once in 3 months for a year and annual mammogram
   c. Regular checking of LFT once in 6 months
   d. Follow-up with Tumor markers once in 6 months
4. **A patient met with a RTA with paralysis of both upper and lower limb. Patient has not passed urine and tenderness elicited in the cervical region. What will you advise?**
   a. The doctor should order a cervical X-ray and shift the patient from the trolley by himself
   b. The patient should not be shifted and portable X-ray machine should be used after neck stabilization
   c. The doctor will instruct the radiographer to take cervical and chest X-ray
   d. The doctor will instruct the radiographer to take cervical X-ray AP and lateral view without any cervical support

5. **A young male with complaints of acute abdominal pain. A plain X-ray abdomen erect was taken which is shown below. Your diagnosis is:**

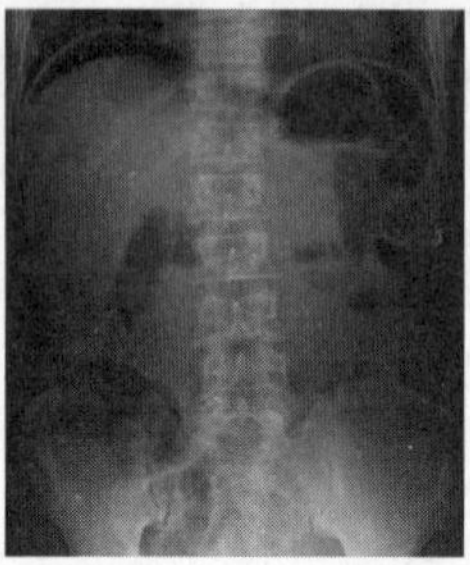

a. Pneumoperitoneum
b. Pneumopericardium
c. Intestinal obstruction
d. Subdiaphragmatic abscess

6. **A person met with an accident and came to casualty with contusion on left precordium. Normal heart sounds are heard but there was decreased breath sounds on left side and trachea deviated to right. Which of the following is the first line of management?**

a. Needle thoracocentesis
b. Chest tube insertion
c. Pericardiocentesis
d. Open surgery

7. **A 24-year-old patient presented with history of neck swelling which moves with deglutition as shown below. Your diagnosis is:**

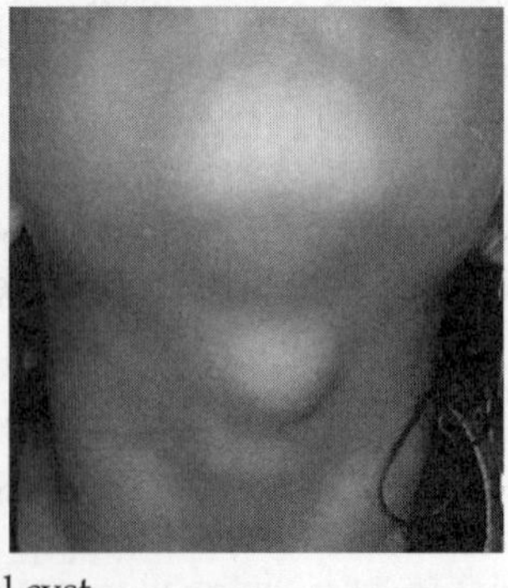

a. Thyroglossal cyst
b. Branchial cyst
c. Cystic hygroma
d. Cervical lymphadenopathy

8. **Which of the following is the flap shown in the picture?**

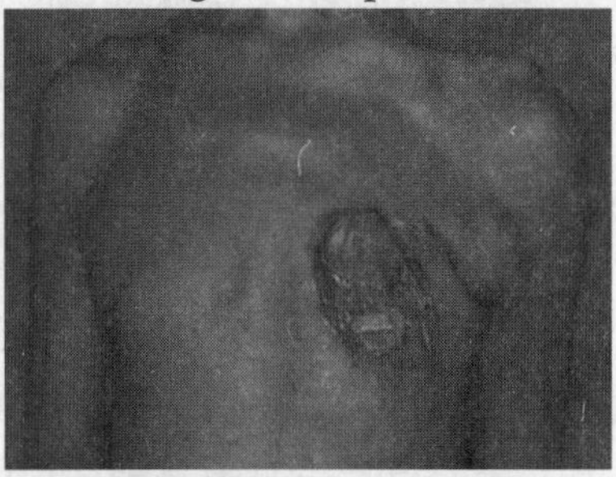

(See Color Plate 10)

a. Serratus anterior flap
b. Pectoral myocutaneous flap
c. TRAM flap
d. VRAM flap

9. **A 30-year-old female with history of burns involving abdomen, both limbs and back and presented after 8 hours. Which of the following is the formula for calculation of fluid infusion?**

a. 4 mL/kg × %TBSA for first 8 hours then 2 mL/kg × %TBSA for next 16 hours
b. 2 mL/kg × %TSBA
c. 4 mL/kg × %TSBA
d. 5 mL/kg ×%TSBA

10. **A 5-year-old boy came to the OPD with scald injury of arm. The lesion was pink, oozing and painful to air and touch. Which of the following is the most appropriate management?**

a. Collagen dressing
b. Paraffin gauze and leave the wound open
c. Excision and grafting
d. Apply 1% silver sulfadiazine

11. **A 30-year-old female was admitted to casualty with history of head trauma in a RTA. Her eye opens to pain, moans, localizes toward the pain on left-hand and away from the pain on right hand, both the legs in extended posture. Calculate her GCS:**

a. 11
b. 3
c. 7
d. 9

12. **A patient presented to the emergency department with fever and pain abdomen. He has history of diarrhea for several months. Abdominal X-ray is shown below. What is the most probable diagnosis?**

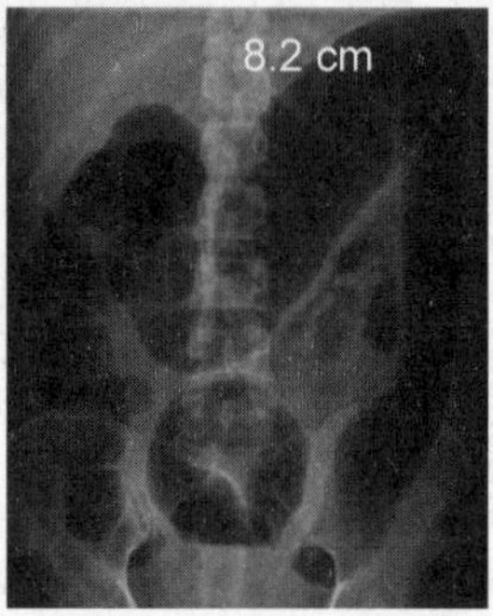

a. Pneumatosis intestinalis
b. Toxic megacolon
c. Volvulus
d. Intestinal perforation

13. A 27-year-old pregnant women came with history of thyroid swelling. FNAC report was suggestive of papillary carcinoma thyroid and the nodule was "cold" on scan. Which of the following will not be a treatment option for her?

a. Radioiodine ablation of thyroid
b. Total thyroidectomy
c. Right hemithyroidectomy
d. Total thyroidectomy plus lymph node dissection

14. A 18-year-old boy presented to the emergency unit with history of fever and abdominal pain. On examination he was febrile and pulse rate was 104/min. The resident was eliciting the sign shown below. Identify the sign.

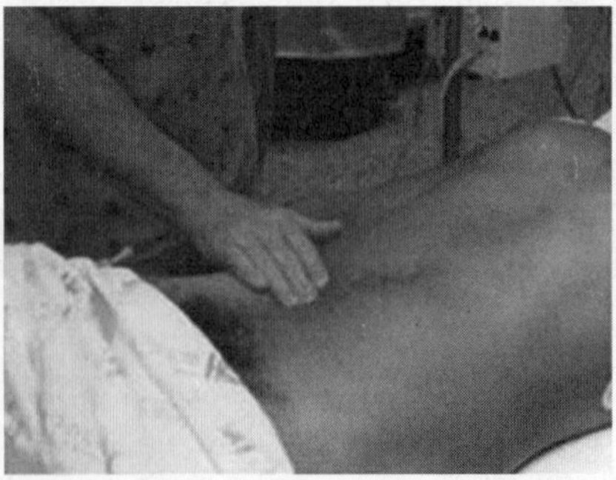

a. Rovsing's sign
b. Ballance sign
c. Blumberg sign
d. Psoas sign

15. A 45-year-old female with H/O painless breast lump presents with a lump 6.4 × 4.3 cm in left upper outer quadrant, no axillary nodes are seen. Core cut biopsy showed Ductal Carcinoma in situ. She undergoes surgery with resection of all tumour tissue with adequate margins and postoperative HPE showed with DCIS with high grade necrosis with 4 mm clearance on margins. Which of the following is needed?

a. Adjuvant chemotherapy
b. Adjuvant radiotherapy
c. Adjuvant chemoradiotherapy
d. No additional treatment

16. A 56-year-old gentleman came to casualty with history of massive hemoptysis. His chest X-ray and other investigation are normal. Which of the following you will not do to prevent hemoptysis?

a. Pulmonary artery embolization
b. Bronchial artery embolization
c. Surgical removal of lobe
d. Procoagulant drugs

17. Pancreatic cancer has the highest association with:

a. Hereditary pancreatitis
b. Peutz-Jeghers syndrome
c. FAP
d. FAMMM syndrome

18. What is the percentage that an USG can detect lymph node metastases in a patient with breast cancer and clinically negative lymph nodes?

a. 10–20%
b. 20–30%
c. 30–50%
d. 50–60%

19. Kraissl's lines are:

a. Point of maximum tension in a fracture
b. Point of tension in hanging
c. Collagen and elastin lines in stab injury
d. Relaxed Tension lines in skin

EXPLANATIONS

1. **Ans. a. Pigtail insertion and drainage**

(Ref. Sabiston Textbook of Surgery, 20th ed; pg1501–1504)

The possible diagnosis in this clinical scenario looks seem to be of bile duct injury, a complication seen post laparoscopic cholecystectomy.

Possible steps to prevent bile duct injuries

- High quality imaging with 30° laparoscope to be preffered
- Firm cephalic traction on fundus and lateral traction on infundibulum, so cystic duct lies perpendicular to CBD
- Dissect at only infundibulocystic junction
- Expose "Critical view of safety" before dividing cystic duct
- Convert to open, if unable to mobilise infundibulum or bleeding or inflammation in Calot's triangle
- Routine intraoperative cholangiogram and Intraoperative laparoscopic ultrasound (IOUS)

Presentation of bile duct injuries

- About 25% recognized intraoperatively
- About 25% discovered within 24 hours postoperative
- About 50% present weeks to years postoperative.
- Most INJURIES are not recognized intraoperatively, and patients are usually sent home
- Patients who fails to recover within first few days or develop progressive vague abdominal symptoms
- Abdominal fullness, distension, nausea, vomiting, abdominal pain, fever and chills
- Symptoms can leads to bilomas, biliary fistula, cholangitis, sepsis, or multi organ system failure
- Clinical presentation:
  - Biliary obstructions leading to anorexia, jaundice, elevated LFT
  - Bile leaks
  - Both can occur simultaneously
  - Concomitant vascular injuries (complicate matter)
- Obstruction secondary to biliary stricture appear weeks to month later and may present with recurrent colangitis, obstructive jaundice, or secondary biliary cirrosis.

MANAGEMENT OF BILE DUCT INJURY AFTER CHOLECYSTECTOMY

Principles of Management

- Control the infection (as bile is an irritant)
- **Control the inflammation by drainage of the collections**
- Wait some months to allow inflammation to heal and fibrosis to settle

- Clear evaluation of the biliary anatomy by Percutaneous Transhepatic Cholangiogram (needed in biliary stricture with IHBR dilatation) or MRCP (almost indicated in all cases) or ERCP
- **Planned Elective Intervention Later on**
- **Primary repair has a high incidence of failure, which may require a percutaneous or endoscopic balloon dilatation later.**

Management Protocol

- Parenteral antibiotics
- **USG guided percutaneous drainage of collections**
- ERCP and Stenting (needed in cases where cystic duct stump leak is suspected) and Imaging to delineate biliary anatomy
- Treatment options: Surgery (based on the **Strasberg classification of bile duct stricture)**
- If there is no 'Tissue Lost', a **primary repair (end to end CBD repair) is preffered** over T-tube, but stricture rate is high!!!
- If there is 'Tissue Lost', **biliodigestive anastomosis** is attempted, choledocoduodenostomy/Roux-en-Y hepaticojejunostomy is attempted.

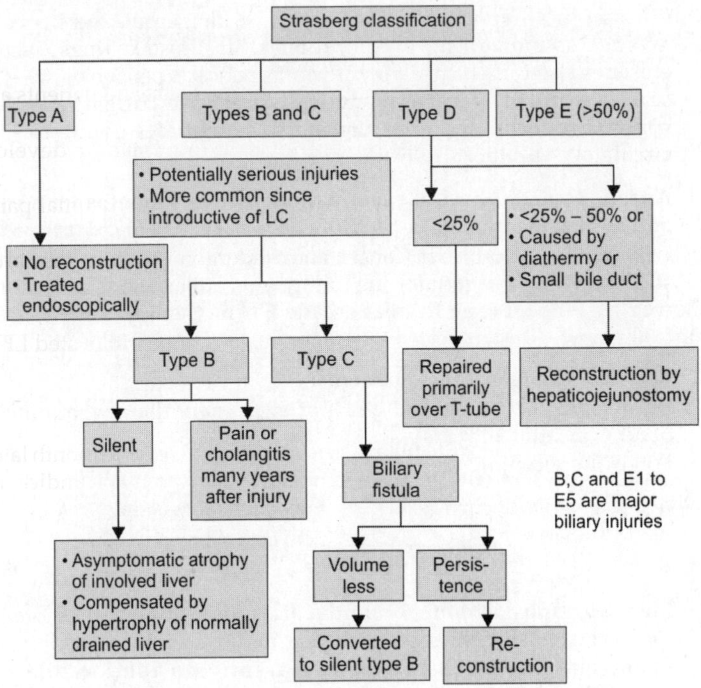

2. **Ans. d. All patients should have chest X-ray – PA view only**

(Ref. Schwartz Principles of Surgery, 10th edition; p161,173)

All trauma patients are managed based on **Advanced Trauma Life Support** guidelines.

- **Steps are**
  - Triage
  - Primary survey
  - Emergency resuscitation
  - Adjuncts to primary survey
  - Secondary survey
  - Adjuncts to secondary survey
- **Primary Survey includes**
  - Airway and cervical spine stabilization
  - Breathing and ventilation
  - Circulation and blood loss control
  - Disability and neurologic evaluation
  - Exposure/Environment
- Imaging of the cervical spine can be done later after complete evaluation of spinal cord injuries
- Patients with blunt trauma are **always sent for plain radiographs of Chest and Pelvis with Anteroposterior Views** as the patient will be in supine position and not PA views.
- CT scan in a hypotensive patient can be dangerous and hence is avoided as monitoring is compromised in those settings, acute episodes also can't be dealt in CT rooms hence as per Schwartz—**CT scan is avoided in hemodynamically unstable patients. Further contrast induced organ damages also potentiates owing to low circulatory volume.**

3. **Ans. b. Routine physical examination once in 3 months for a year and annual mammogram** *(Ref. Bailey and Love, 26th edition; p816)*

The patient has Early Breast Cancer and undergone surgery probably Breast conservation Surgery for the Lump and Axillary nodal dissection followed by Whole Breast Irradiation and Chemotherapy. Patient is on Tamoxifen now.

FOLLOW-UP of breast cancer patients:

- **Recurrences occur within 5 years after primary therapy**, but it can occur even after 20 years.
- Following recommendations are followed:

Every 3–6 months	**For years 1 through 3**
Every 6–12 months	For years 4 through 5
Annually	After 5 years

- **Mammography is done 6 months** after the completion of **Breast Conservation surgery** and after a year in those with mastectomy.
- Bailey and Love says **"There is currently no routine role for repeated measurements of tumor markers or imaging other than mammography"**

4. **Ans. b. The patient should not be shifted and portable X-ray machine should be used after neck stabilization**

(Ref. Sabiston Textbook of Surgery, 20th edition; p420-421)

Management of Cervical Spine Injury in a Trauma Patient:

- The spine should always be immobilized assuming a spine injury until proven otherwise
- Blunt and penetrating trauma result in different forms of spinal cord injury.
  - Blunt trauma causes cord injury through direct impingement or indirect compression due to vertebral fracture or dislocation.
  - Penetrating trauma causes direct cord laceration or indirectly through ischemia or fracture.
- Following steps are followed:

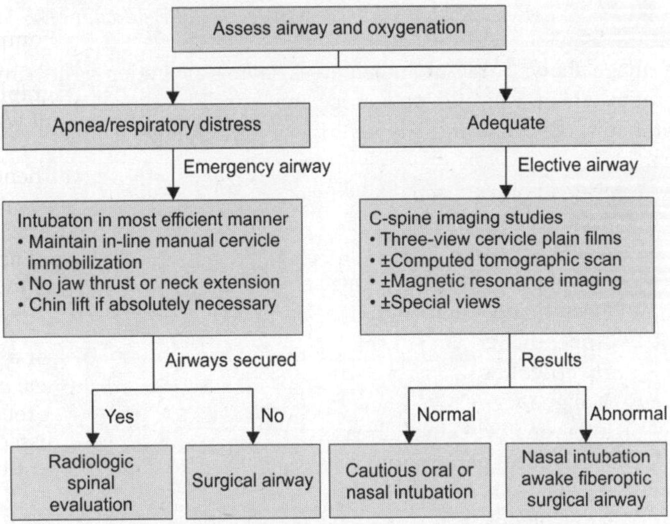

- Spine immobilization done and after immobilization X-ray attempted with a portable machine

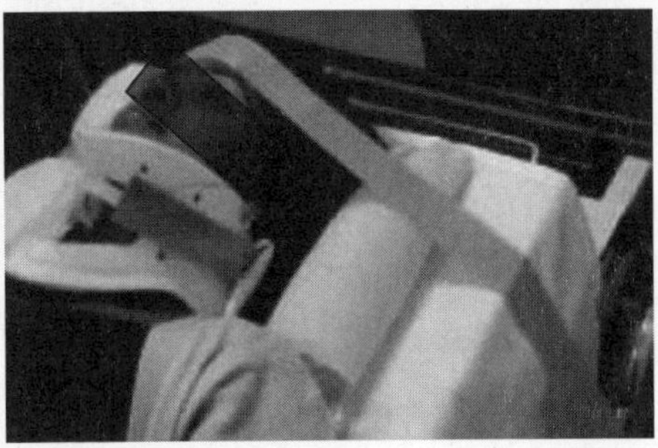

- X-rays in the acute trauma are usually taken with the help of portable X-ray machine which includes AP views of cervical, chest and pelvis, as unnecessary mobilization and shifting of the patient might aggravate injury even with immobilization by cervical collar.

EXTRA EDGE:

- Spine surgeon opinion should be obtained
- Patients with neurogenic shock should be given volume expansion and
- **Corticosteroids** previously considered useful, nowadays **considered ineffective.**

5. Ans. a. Pneumoperitoneum

(Ref. Sabiston Textbook of Surgery, 20th edition; p1126-1128)

The image shows X-ray abdomen erect having air under right hemidiaphragm which indicates pneumoperitoneum. The causes of pneumoperitoneum are wide and the severity of accompanying illness is also variable:

- Perforated hollow viscus
  - Peptic ulcer disease
  - Ischemic bowel
  - Bowel obstruction
  - Necrotizing enterocolitis
  - Appendicitis
  - Diverticulitis
  - Malignancy
  - Inflammatory bowel disease
  - Mechanical perforation
    - Trauma
    - Colonoscopy
    - Foreign bodies
    - Iatrogenic
- Postoperative free intraperitoneal gas
- Peritoneal dialysis
- Vaginal "aspiration"
  - Cunnilingus
  - Douching
  - Sudden squatting
  - Postpartum exercises
- Mechanical ventilation
- Pneumomediastinum
- Pneumothorax.

Radiological Signs on X-ray

- **Bowel-related signs**
  - Double wall sign (Rigler's sign or bas-relief sign)
  - Telltale triangle sign (also known as triangle sign)
- **Peritoneal ligament-related signs**
  - Football sign
  - Falciform ligament sign
  - Lateral umbilical ligament sign (also known as inverted "V" sign)
  - Urachus sign
- **Right upper quadrant signs**
  - Lucent liver sign
  - Hepatic edge sign
  - Fissure for ligamentum teres sign
  - Morison's pouch sign (doge cap sign)
  - Cupola sign.

6. Ans. b. Chest tube insertion

(Ref. Schwartz Principles of Surgery, 10th edition; p163-164)

The clinical picture here of Blunt trauma to the chest with normal vitals, decreased breath sounds on left side with tracheal deviation to right gives a diagnosis of pneumothorax.

Shift of trachea and diminished sounds indicate moderate pneumothorax, the ideal management of this scenario is chest tube insertion.

Only small apical pneumothorax < 25% can be attempted to manage conservatively of with a needle thoracocentesis.

- Management of simple pneumothorax includes chest tube insertion **or Tube thoracostomy inserted at the Triangle of safety**, which is bounded by lateral border of pectoralis major anteriorly, Latissimus dorsi posteriorly and inferiorly by an imaginary line drawn at the level of nipple, i.e. 5th ICS.

7. Ans. a. Thyroglossal cyst

(Ref: Sabiston Textbook of Surgery, 20th edition; p1861)

Short Cases in Surgery by Das, pg. 100 – 111.

- Thyroglossal duct cysts account for 70% of all congenital neck anomalies, and are the second most common benign neck mass, after lymphadenopathy.

The **swellings that moves up with deglutition are as follows:**

- **Thyroid swellings**
- **Ectopic thyroid**
- **Thyroglossal cyst**

- **Subhyoid bursal cyst**
- **Enlarged pretracheal nodes which are fixed to trachea**
- **Laryngocele**

The cysts can occur anywhere along the course of the thyroglossal duct, although infrahyoid location is most common:

- Suprahyoid: 20–25% (less common in adults 5%)
- At the level of hyoid bone: 30% (range 15–50%)
- Infrahyoid: 45% (range 25–65%)

Typically, they are located in the midline (~70%) with those off-midline characteristically tucked next to the thyroid cartilage. Almost all thyroglossal duct cysts are located within 2 cm of the midline, with more inferior lesions tending to be off midline.

8. Ans. a. Serratus anterior flap

(Ref: Schwartz Principles of Surgery, 10th edition; p1872-1875)

The picture shows a flap reconstruction of the chest wall using serratus anterior myocutaneous flap with skin graft as it involves reconstruction of lower chest wall.

- **Reconstructive options include**
  - Pectoral myocutaneous flap – used in upper chest and midline wounds
  - Transverse Rectus Abdominis Myocutaneous flap (TRAM) – used to cover larger area
  - Vertical Rectus Abdominis Myocutaneous flap (VRAM) – better vascular supply
  - Latissimus dorsi flap with serratus anterior flap – more commonly used to cover nonsternal chest wall defects, mostly in the lower chest wall.

Latissimus serratus anterior flap:

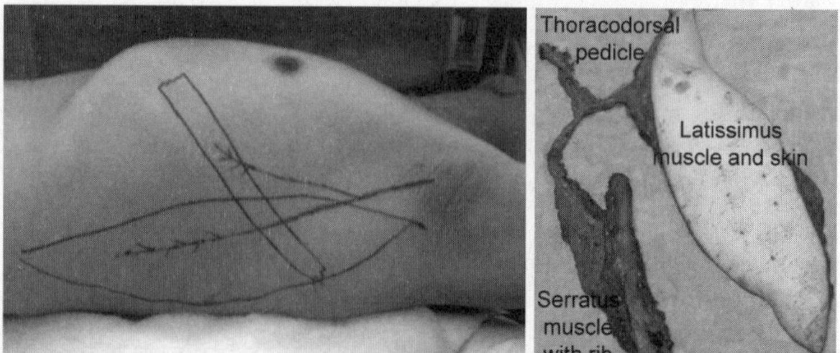

TRAM flap:

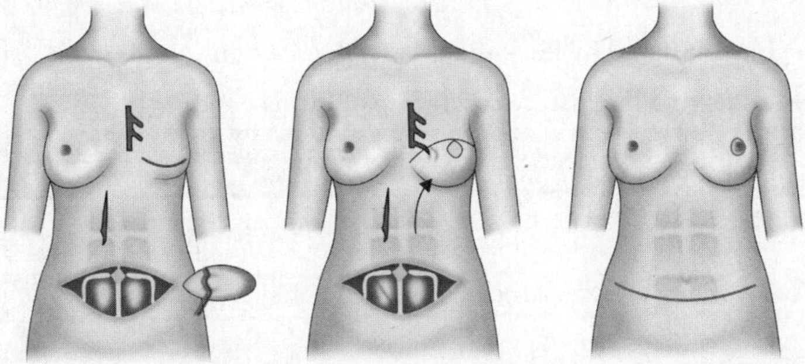

9. **Ans. c. 4 mL/kg × %TSBA**

(Ref: Bailey and Love, 26th edition; p390-392)

- **Indications for fluid resuscitation are**
  - **In adults when the Total Burnt Surface Area is more than 15%**
  - **In children when the Total Burnt Surface Area is more than 10%**
- The Initial rate of infusion is calculated by the following formula
  - % TBSA × Wt(kg)/8
- The amount of liters of fluid generated from formula should be divided into half; **half of which is given in first 8 hours and another half in next 16 hours.**

Name and use	Formula
Parkland or Baxter formula (ADULTS) Use for Crystalloid infusion	4 mL × Wt(kg) x %TBSA
Muir and Barclay formula Use for colloid infusion	0.5 mL × Wt(kg) × %TBSA = 1 part This 1 part is given every 4/4/4 hours, then every 6/6 hours and 12 hours.
Brooke formula (Crystalloid)	1.5 mL × Wt(kg) × %TBSA
Brooke formula (Colloid)	0.5 mL × Wt(kg) × %TBSA
Galveston formula (CHILDREN)	5000 mL/TBSA (in m^2) + 1500 mL/Total body surface area in m^2

- The basis to monitor fluid resuscitation is urine output.
  - **In adults, it should be more than 0.5 mL/hour and in children, more than 1 mL/hour**.
  - If the urine output is below this, the infusion rate should be increased by 50%.

First option will be practically harmful, it should have been 2 mL/kg/TBSA in first 8 hours and 2 mL/kg/TBSA in next 16 hours. Because, over resuscitation should be avoided to prevent massive edema overall and increased risk of compartment syndrome and pulmonary edema.

10. Ans. b. Paraffin gauze and leave the wound open

(Ref: Bailey and Love, 26th edition; p392-394)

The burn suffered by the patient is 1st degree burn.

Table showing the features of degree of burns depth

First degree	Superficial second	Deep second degree	Third degree
Painful	Painful	Painful only to pin prick	**Painless**
Erythematous	Erythematous	Pale and mottled	**Hard leathery eschar**
Blanch to touch	Blanch to touch	Not blanch	Black in color
Not Blister	**BLISTER**		
No scarring	Spontaneous re-epithelialization in 1–2 weeks	Severe scarring and re-epithelialize in 2–5 weeks	**Excision and Skin grafting needed**

WOUND CARE GUIDELINES BASED ON THE BURNS DEPTH

First degree	Topical soothing agents, leave wound open
Superficial second degree	Needs daily dressing
Deep second degree	Excision and grafting
Third degree	Escharotomy and serial excision with grafting

- The various dressings and antimicrobial salves and soaks include
  - 1% **silver sulfadiazine (easy to use, painless**, but does not penetrate eschar)
  - **Mafenide acetate (painful, but penetrates eschar, cause metabolic acidosis)**
  - Mupirocin
  - Polymyxin B, Bacitracin, Neomycin
  - Dakin solution (0.25% sodium hypochlorite)
  - 0.5% silver nitrate solution
  - 0.25% acetic acid solution
  - Hydrocolloid dressings
  - Permeable wound dressing like Mefix and Fixamull.

11. Ans. d. 9

(Ref: Bailey and Love, 26th edition; p312)

The female has sustained a trauma to the head and her GCS response is given. The calculation will be:

- Eye opening to pain is E2

- Moaning is V2
- Localizes towards pain on left is M5 and withdrawal on right is M4
- Total score will be E2 V2 M5 = 9

Value	Motor response	Verbal response	Eye response
6	Moves all 4 limbs		
5	Localizes pain	Oriented	
4	Withdraws to painful stimuli	Confused	Eye opened
3	Flexor or Decorticate response	Inappropriate words	Opens to verbal commands
2	Extensor (Decerebrate) response	Incomprehensible sounds	Opens to painful stimuli
1	No response	No response	No response

12. Ans. b. Toxic megacolon

(Ref: Schwartz Principles of Surgery, 10th edition; p1197-98)

The patient in question has acute abdominal pain associated with fever and history of diarrhea several months coupled with the image findings showing Dilated entire colon with loss of haustrations with diameter about 8.2 cm – all pointing toward Toxic Megacolon in a patient with Ulcerative Colitis.

- **Toxic Megacolon is an extreme dilation of the colon in which the affected area of bowel loses all tone and contractility**. Bowel sounds, peristalsis, and bowel movements cease. The patient will have progressive abdominal distension, significant discomfort, fever, and often leukocytosis.

Ruling out other options:

1. Intestinal perforation is associated with peritonitis and gas under diaphragm in X-ray
2. Volvulus is axial rotation or twisting of a portion of a bowel about its own axis at the site of attachment. It is common in Sigmoid colon and also cecum, which are mobile parts. It has a characteristic bent tyre tube sign, with concavity facing toward the pelvis to the left.
3. **Pneumatosis intestinalis is characterized by intramural bowel gas, i.e., gas within the bowel wall** as it is seen in cases of necrotizing enterocolitis, mesenteric ischemia where the gangrenous bowel impart this feature due to gas producing microorganisms.

13. Ans. a. Radioiodine ablation of thyroid

(Ref: Sabiston Textbook of Surgery, 20th edition; p903-908; Bailey and Love, 26th edition; p766-768)

Radioiodine ablation is contraindicated during pregnancy as it causes increased radiation risk to the fetus.

- More common in females,
- Between the ages 3rd and 4th decade
- It has **rich intrathyroidal lymphatic network and hence higher chance of multifocal** involvement in the thyroid gland
- It has higher incidence of nodal metastases
- Generally, thyroid cancers have nodal **metastases in the pretracheal, paratracheal and prelaryngeal (Delphian) nodes in the Central Compartment, i.e. Level VI.**
- Mostly papillary carcinoma presents as a solitary nodule, which is firm in consistency.
- It can cause hoarseness by invasion of recurrent laryngeal nerve.
- USG neck and thyroid shows an **irregular hypoechogenic solid lesion with rich intranodal vascularity and microcalcifications**.
- The lesion will be taller than wide on transverse view of the sonography probe.
- The diagnosis is easily established by doing USG guided FNA of the suspicious nodule, which shows **pseudonuclear inclusions, nuclear ingrooving giving an Orphan Annie Eye appearance. There are also psammoma bodies** which are concretions of dead and necrotic tissue that present with dystrophic calcification.
- Once the diagnosis of papillary carcinoma has been made, patient should have **USG neck to rule out any nodal metastases and look for invasion of nodule to adjacent structures to stage the disease**.
- No need for CECT neck.
- Patient evaluated to have clinically node negative, should undergo total thyroidectomy alone and those who have central compartment nodes should undergo an additional central compartmental neck dissection
- Overall papillary carcinoma carries a relatively good prognosis with a 20 year survival rate of ~90%. The 5-year survival is in the range of 95%.
- If the tumor is confined to the gland then mortality is less than 2.5%, with a sharp increase in mortality in patients with extension beyond the gland, to 38%.

14. Ans. c. Blumberg sign

(Ref: Bailey and Love, 26th edition; p1202-1203)

The patient has abdominal pain and is febrile and tachycardiac.

The picture shows eliciting tenderness at the McBurney's point which is located at a point situated between lateral one-third and medial two-thirds of the right spinoumbilical line, causing tenderness in the setting of acute appendicitis.

SIGNS IN ACUTE APPENDICITIS

Pointing sign	Patient points the McBurney's point using finger
McBurney tenderness	Pain in RIF at McBurney's point
Blumberg's release sign	Rebound tenderness due to parietal peritonitis
Rovsing's sign	Indirect tenderness in RIF, by pressing in LIF
Dunphy's sign	Pain during coughing
Cope psoas test	Lateral decubitus, extension of hip (retrocecal appendix)
Cope obturator test	Internal rotation of flexed thigh (Pelvic appendix)
Aaron sign	Pain or pressure in epigastrium or anterior chest with persistent firm pressure applied to McBurney's point
Ten Horn sign	Pain caused by gentle traction of right testicle

15. Ans. d. No additional treatment

(Ref: Sabiston Textbook of Surgery, 20th edition; p851-855, NCCN Guidelines for Breast Cancer; DCIS)

- The patient in question is a middle-aged female had breast lump 6.2 × 4.5 cm without nodes diagnosed to be DCIS for which surgery done (probably simple mastectomy considering the size of the tumour and the cosmetic outcome following wide local excision if done; read the indications for Mastectomy in DCIS below).
- HPE came out has DCIS with high grade necrosis with 4 mm clearance margins. **No additional treatment needed following Mastectomy.**
- Had the question given Wide local excision or lumpectomy (in such case, it is considered a wrongly framed question), which is not possible for such a huge lump, the next step will be Radiotherapy to prevent the recurrence as high grade DCIS with narrow margins tend to recur.
- **No role for chemotherapy in DCIS** as it is noninvasive breast cancer.

DUCTAL CARCINOMA IN SITU

- DCIS is an **anatomic precursor of Invasive ductal carcinoma**
- Epithelial proliferation in the minor ducts resulting in papillary growth **(papillary growth pattern)**. Later these coalesce and fill the lumina so that only scattered round spaces remain **(cribriform growth pattern).**
- Eventually they obliterate the lumen and distend the ducts **(solid growth pattern).** With continued growth, cells become necrotic **(Comedo)** and calcium deposition occurs **(microcalcification in mammography)**
- Classification of DCIS

Histologic type	Nuclear grade	Necrosis	DCIS grade
Comedo	High	Extensive	High
Intermediate	Intermediate	Focal	Intermediate
Non Comedo	Low	Absent	Low

MANAGEMENT OF DUCTAL CARCINOMA IN SITU

- Treatment options are **BCS (Breast Conservation Surgery) / BCS with WBRT (50 Gy) / Mastectomy + Tamoxifen (ER +ve)**
- **Axillary dissection and chemotherapy are not needed**
- But Sentinel Lymph Node Biopsy has a role if Mastectomy is planned, as there is **20% incidence of invasive BC on final pathologic assessment of primary tumor.**
- Several studies and data said that selected patients with DCIS might not require postoperative RT as there was no benefit when the margins are more than 10 mm.

Silverstein – Van Nuy's Prognostic Index for DCIS

Parameteres	Score 1	Score 2	Score 3
Size	</= 1.5 cm	1.6 to 4 cm	> 4 cm
Margin	>/= 10 mm	1 to 9 mm	<1 mm
Class	Grade 1 or 2 without necrosis	Grade 1 or 2 with necrosis	Grade 3
Age	>60	40–60	<40

- Scores 4, 5, 6, 7 with >3 mm margin → Excision alone
- **Scores 7 with < 3 mm margin, 8 with > 3 mm margin, 9 with >5 mm margin → Excision + RT**
- Score 9 with < 5 mm margin, 10, 11, 12 → Mastectomy

Indications for mastectomy in DCIS:
Extensive DCIS component (> 4 cm)
Multicentric
Poor cosmetic outcome and not willing to preserve breast
Contraindications for BCS (Prior irradiation)
Contraindications for RT (Pregnancy, Collagen vascular diseases)
Failure to get clear margins after BCS 2 times

16. **Ans. d. Procoagulant drugs**

(Ref: Schwartz Principles of Surgery, 10th edition; p662)

"Management of Massive hemoptysis doesn't includes use of Procoagulant drugs"

- **600 mL of expectoration within 24 hours constitute massive**
- Acute Emergency with a mortality rate of 30% to 50%.
- **Common causes for massive hemoptysis** are
  - Pulmonary cancer
  - Pulmonary trauma
  - Bronchiectasis
  - Tuberculosis
  - Pulmonary embolism

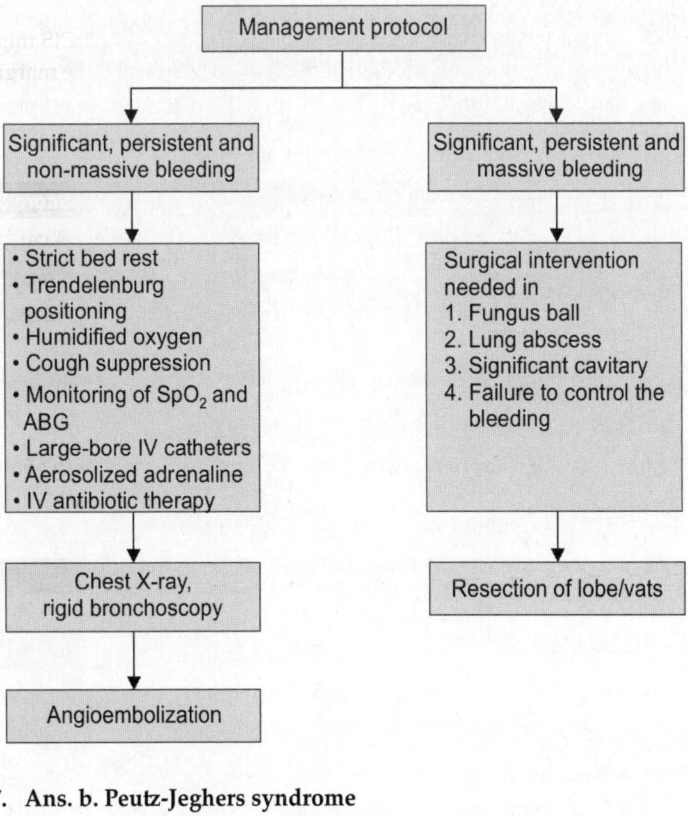

17. **Ans. b. Peutz-Jeghers syndrome**

(Ref: Sabiston Textbook of Surgery, 20th edition; p1541-1543)

Risk factors

Name	Defect	Risk of pancreatic cancer
Peutz-Jeghers syndrome	**STK11 gene mutation**	**100 fold increased risk**
Hereditary Pancreatitis	**Mutation in cationic trypsinogen PRSS1 gene**	**50 fold increased risk**
Cystic Fibrosis	**CFTR gene mutation**	**30 fold increased risk**
FAMMM syndrome	**CDKN2A gene mutation**	**20 fold increased risk**
Hereditary breast and ovarian cancer	BRCA 2 gene mutation	10 fold increased risk
Lynch syndrome	MLH1 gene mutation	8 fold increased risk
FAP	**APC gene mutation**	**4 fold increased risk**
Familial pancreatic cancer	Unknown gene	18 fold increased risk

18. Ans. d. 50–60%

(Ref: Schwartz Principles of Surgery, 10th edition; p527,531)

- Suspicious signs of nodal metastasis
  - Cortical thickening
  - Absence of hilum or decrease in size
  - Changes in shape or vascular pattern
  - Increase in size more than 10 mm and
  - Hypoechoic echoes

➢ Accuracy of axillary ultrasound in detecting lymph node metastases in patients with breast cancer,

Sensitivity	47.6%
Specificity	95.7%
Positive predictive value	85.9%
Negative predictive Vale	77%
Accuracy of axillary USG	78.7%

19. Ans. d. Relaxed Tension lines in skin

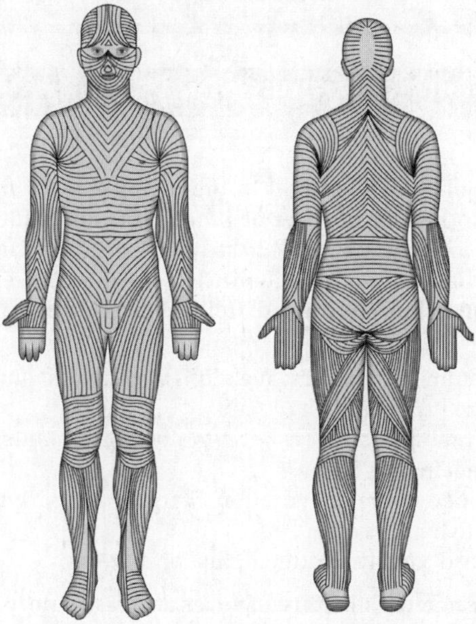

(Ref: Grays Anatomy Chapter 7, 41/e p157)

- Kraissl's lines are oriented perpendicular to the action of the underlying muscles
- Kraissl's lines coincides with wrinkle lines, and tend to be perpendicular to the muscle action
- Kraissl's lines are found by studying the direction of underlying muscle fiber
- Kraissl transposed wrinkle lines over diagrams of the underlying musculature and showed that these lines are mostly perpendicular to the muscles
- Collagen runs generally parallel to wrinkle lines and is laid down parallel to scars
- In a scar placed perpendicular to the underlying muscle, collagen will be laid down in the same direction as is usual in the wrinkle lines and the septa between skin and muscle
- **Borges's and Kraissl's lines are better guides for elective incisions in the face and body, respectively**, than Langer's lines.

PEDIATRICS

QUESTIONS

1. **A 5-year-old child brought to the hospital with history of loose stools. No history of fever or blood in stools. Mother says he is irritable and drinks water hastily when given. On examination eyes are sunken and in Skin pinch test—the skin retracted within two seconds but not immediately. What is the treatment for this child?**
   a. IV administer the first dose of IV antibiotic and immediately refer to higher center
   b. Give oral fluids and ask the mother to continue the same and visit again next day
   c. Consider severe dehydration. Start IV fluids, IV antibiotics and refer to higher center
   d. No need for any treatment. Just observe

2. **A child came with history of fever and respiratory distress. With a suspicion of pneumonia, chest X-ray was ordered. Which of the following is most likely organism?**

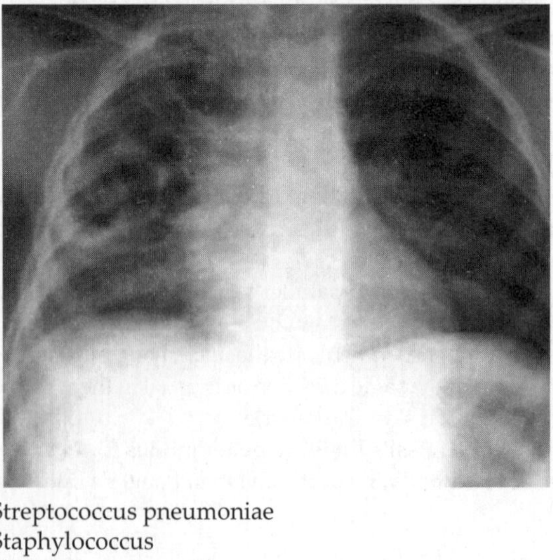

   a. Streptococcus pneumoniae
   b. Staphylococcus
   c. Klebsiella pneumoniae
   d. Mycoplasma pneumoniae

3. **Which of the following is true regarding congenital CMV infection?**
   a. Diagnosed only by persistent presence of IgM antibody after 6 months
   b. It's the most common cause on nonsyndromic sensory neural hearing loss
   c. All babies born are symptomatic
   d. Mothers of developing countries who transmit the virus are usually symptomatic

4. **Which of the following is not seen in fetal alcohol syndrome?**
   a. Microcephaly
   b. Macrocephaly
   c. Thinning of corpus callosum
   d. Holoprosencephaly

5. **An 18-month-old child brought to the hospital with history of breathlessness, fever, cough and cold. On examination respiratory rate was 49/min, there were no chest retractions. Which is the most appropriate management?**
   a. Give IV antibiotics and refer to higher center
   b. Oral antibiotics, warn of danger signs and send home
   c. IV antibiotics and observe
   d. No need of treatment. Only home remedies

6. **A 14-day neonate had conjunctivitis, which later developed into respiratory distress and pneumonia. Chest X-ray showed bilateral lung infiltrates. Peripheral smear count showed 14,800/dL (N 43, L 54, E3). Which of the following is the most likely organism?**
   a. Streptococcus agalactiae
   b. Mycoplasma pneumoniae
   c. Neisseria gonorrhoeae
   d. Chlamydia trachomatis

EXPLANATIONS

1. Ans. b. Give oral fluids and ask the mother to continue the same and visit again next day *(Ref: IMNCI Protocol)*

Let's approach the question systematically with the **"art of finding keywords"**. As hinted by the examiner:

- We are expected to predict the degree of dehydration first
- The child's mental status → Normal, fatigued or restless, **irritable**
- Thirst → **Thirsty and eager to drink**
- Eyes → **Sunken**
- Skinfold → **Recoil in < 2 sec** (but NOT instantly, hence NOT minimal/ no dehydration).

So from these keywords, we can conclude that the child has = **Mild to Moderate Dehydration (3–9% Loss of Body Weight).** Next task is to think of the management plan.

The ideal treatment plan for mild to moderate dehydration according to Nelson 20/E is:

- **Rehydration therapy** = ORS → 50–100 mL/kg body weight over 3–4 hr
- **Replacement of losses** =
  - ***<10 kg body weight: 60–120 mL ORS for each diarrheal stool or vomiting episode***
  - ***>10 kg body weight: 120–240 mL ORS for each diarrheal stool or vomiting episode***
- **Nutrition** = Resume age-appropriate normal diet after initial hydration, including adequate caloric intake for maintenance.

Extra Edge

Tabular key to find the correct degree of dehydration:

Signs and symptoms	Minimal or no dehydration	Mild to moderate dehydration	Severe dehydration
Body weight loss	Less than 3%	6–9%	10% or more
Mental status	Well appearing, alert	Normal, fatigued or restless, or irritable	Apathetic, lethargic, may be unconscious
Thirst	Drinks normally, might refuse liquids	Thirsty, eager to drink	Drinks poorly or unable to drink
Heart rate	Normal	Normal to increased	Increased, might be decreased in more severe cases
Blood pressure	Normal	Normal	Normal to decreased

Contd...

Contd...

Signs and symptoms	Minimal or no dehydration	Mild to moderate dehydration	Severe dehydration
Quality of pulses	Normal	Normal to decreased	Weak, thready, or impalpable
Capillary refill	Normal	± 2 sec	> 3 sec
Respiration	Normal	Normal, might be rapid	Deep and rapid
Eyes	Normal	Slightly sunken	Grossly sunken
Tears	Present	Decreased	Absent
Mucous membranes	Moist	Dry	Very dry
Skin turgor	Instant recoil	Recoil in 2 < sec	Recoil in > 2 sec
Extremities	Warm	Cool	Cold, mottled, cyanotic
Urine output	Normal to decreased	Decreased	Minimal

Treatment plan for dehydration in pediatrics age group:

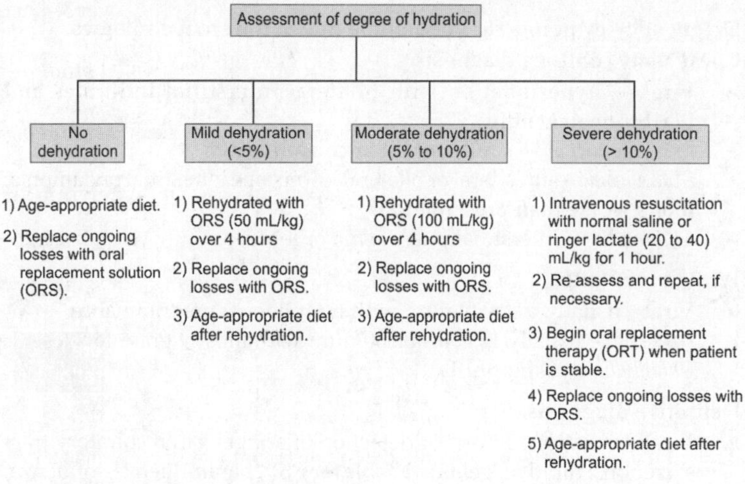

2. **Ans. b. Staphylococcus**

(Ref: Nelson Textbook of Pediatrics, 20/e p2090)

- **The X-ray image shows thin-walled, air-filled cysts developing within the lung parenchyma known as "Pneumatoceles".**
- Pneumatoceles can be single emphysematous lesions but are more often multiple, thin-walled, air-filled, cyst-like cavities.
- Most often, they occur as a **sequela to → acute pneumonia**.

- **Most Commonly** caused by → ***Staphylococcus aureus***. But NOT specific.
- Also occurs with → *Streptococcus pneumoniae, Haemophilus influenzae, Escherichia coli,* Group A streptococci, *Serratia marcescens, Klebsiella pneumoniae,* Adenovirus and tuberculosis.

Image-based Questions Section:

- The image below gives a further clearer idea of the pneumatoceles and other differential diagnoses.

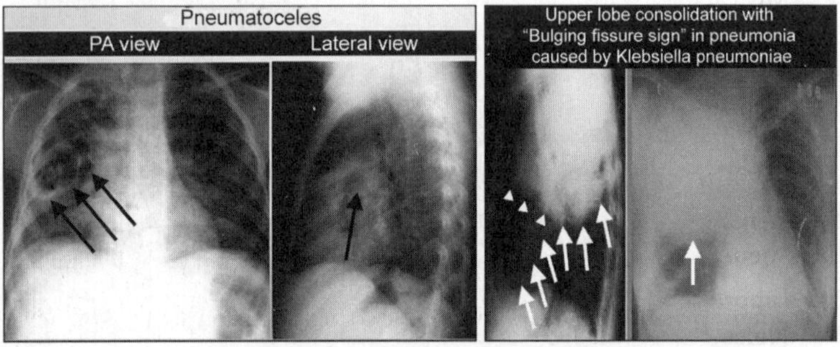

Diagnostic key points for pneumonia due to different etiologies:

Chest X-ray confirms diagnosis:

- Viral → **hyperinflation with bilateral interstitial infiltrates and peribronchial cuffing**
- Pneumococcal → **confluent lobar consolidation**
- *Mycoplasma* → unilateral or bilateral lower-lobe interstitial pneumonia; **looks worse than presentation.**
- *Chlamydia* → interstitial pneumonia or lobar; as with *Mycoplasma*

White blood cells:

- Viral = usually < 20,000/mm^3 with lymphocyte predominance
- Bacterial = usually 15,000–40,000/mm^3 with mostly granulocytes
- *Chlamydia* = **eosinophilia**

Definitive diagnosis:

- Viral = isolation of virus or detection of antigens in respiratory tract secretions; rapid reagents available for RSV, parainfluenza, influenza, and adenovirus
- Bacterial = isolation of organism from blood (positive in only 10–30% of children with *S. pneumoniae*), pleural fluid, or lung; **sputum cultures are of no value in children.** For mycoplasma get IgM titers.

Extra Edge and Potential MCQs on Pneumonia in Pediatric Age Group:

- **Viruses are predominant cause of pneumonia in infants and children < 5 yrs age.**

[MC pathogen is = **RSV** > parainfluenza, influenza, adenovirus]

- **Nonviral causes** more common in **children > 5 years**

  [MC agent is = ***M. pneumoniae*** and ***C. pneumoniae***

  S. pneumoniae is MC with focal infiltrate in children of all ages

  Others in normal children = *S. pyogenes* and *S. aureus* (no longer Hib)
- MC cause for lobar bacterial pneumonia → *S. pneumoniae*
- **Noninfectious causes** of Pneumatoceles → Hydrocarbon ingestion, trauma, positive pressure ventilation.
- MC cause of pneumatoceles in **premature infants with respiratory distress syndrome → ventilator-induced lung injury.**
- **Rx** → Antibiotic treatment of the underlying pneumonia is the first-line therapy. Close observation in the early stages of the infection and periodic follow-up care until resolution of the pneumatocele is usually adequate treatment.

3. **Ans. b. It's the most common cause on nonsyndromic sensory neural hearing loss** *(Ref: Nelson Textbook of Pediatrics, 20/e p1592)*

Let's approach with the "art of ruling out incorrect options":

- **Nelson 20/E writes** – "Congenital infection with CMV can present with **symptomatic infections in approx. 10% of infected newborns,** whereas 90% will have no clinical manifestations of infection in the newborn period." So Option "c" is ruled out.
- "The diagnosis of congenital CMV infections requires the recovery of replicating virus and/or viral nucleic acids **within the 1st 3 weeks of life**." So Option "a" is ruled out.
- **MC long-term sequela associated with congenital CMV infection = Hearing loss,** hence the failure of an infant to pass a newborn hearing screening exam should raise the possibility of congenital CMV infection.
- Hearing loss in the older infant and young child should also alert the clinician to the possibility of congenital CMV infection, as approx. 50% of infants with hearing loss associated with congenital CMV infection will pass an initial hearing screening exam but develop hearing loss in later infancy and early childhood.
- **Hearing loss will develop in = approx. 11% of infected infants** and in some infants hearing loss will progress during infancy. Thus, **audiologic testing and follow-up are mandatory** in these patients. So we can conclude that Option "b" is correct.
- **Transmission:** Women can pass CMV to their baby during pregnancy. The virus in the woman's blood can cross through the placenta and infect the baby. This can occur when a pregnant woman experiences a first-time infection, a reinfection with a different CMV strain (variety),

or a reactivation of a previous infection during pregnancy. Mothers may remain asymptomatic for the infection.

- **Perinatal infections can be acquired during birth or following ingestion of CMV-containing breast milk.**

Extra Edge on Cytomegalovirus (CMV) Infection

- Primary infection (higher risk of severe disease) or reactivation of CMV

Findings:

- Hepatosplenomegaly, jaundice
- **Periventricular calcifications**[Q]
- **Intrauterine growth retardation**[Q]
- **Chorioretinitis**[Q]
- **Microcephaly**[Q]
- Thrombocytopenia, hemolytic anemia

Outcomes:

- **Sensorineural hearing loss**[Q]
- Neuromuscular abnormalities
- Mental retardation

4. **Ans. b. Macrocephaly** *(Ref: Nelson Textbook of Pediatrics, 20/e p895)*

Fetal Alcohol Syndrome (FAS):

- High levels of alcohol ingestion during pregnancy can be damaging to embryonic and fetal development
- Most Common teratogen to which fetus can be exposed is → Alcohol
- Findings are variable:
  - **Symmetric IUGR and postnatal growth deficiency (short stature)**
  - **Mental retardation, microcephaly**[Q]
  - Fine motor dysfunction
  - Irritability in infancy, **hyperactivity in childhood**
  - Behavioral abnormalities
  - **Mid-face dysmorphism** (abnormal frontal lobe development), short palpebral fissures, maxillary hypoplasia, short nose, smooth philtrum, thin and smooth upper lip[Q]
  - **Joint abnormalities**—abnormal position and/or function
  - **Cardiac anomalies: VSD > ASD**, Tetralogy of Fallot
- Macrocephaly is NOT a feature of FAS.

Image-based Questions Section:

- To make the fastest diagnosis in time bound MCQs, look for → short palpebral fissures; long, smooth philtrum with vermillion border; and hirsutism in the newborn.

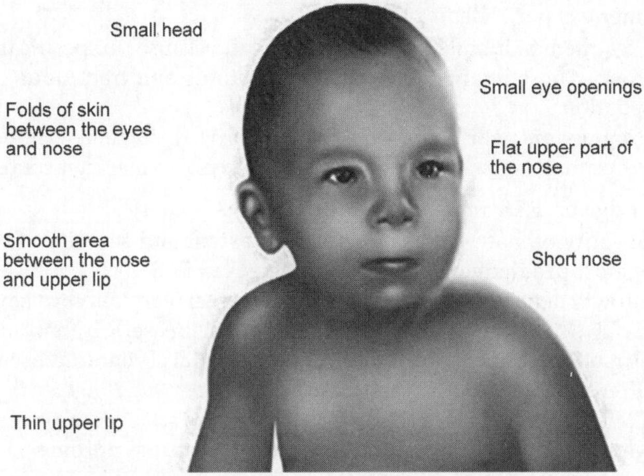

How alcohol affects the developing brain

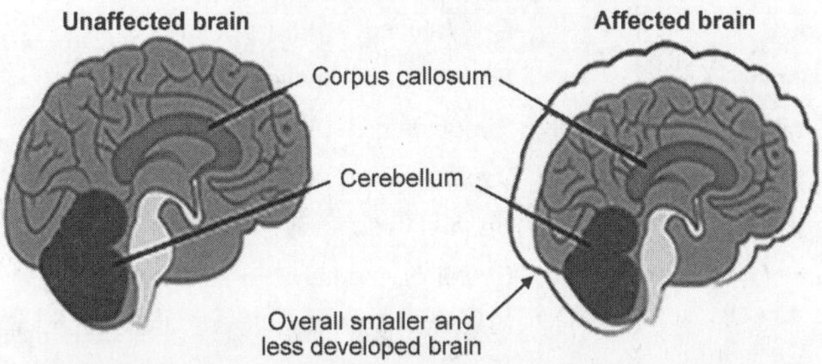

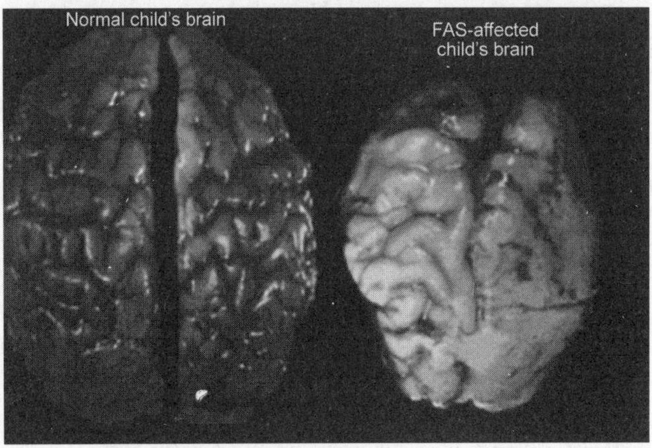

Treatment as per Nelson 20/E:

- Treatment of infants with FAS is difficult because no specific therapy exists. These infants may remain **hypotonic and tremulous** despite sedation.
- **Prognosis is poor:** Counseling with regard to recurrence is important. Prevention is achieved by eliminating alcohol intake after conception.

Extra Edge on FAS and Related Congenital Anomalies:

- **Severity** of maternal alcohol use and **extent and severity of pattern** is **most predictive** of ultimate prognosis in FAS.
- Growth deficiency, borderline to mild mental retardation, dysmorphic facial features, short neck, abnormal palmar crease, Rib abnormalities, **Hirsutism, Cupid's-bow lips** suggest → **Fetal Hydantoin Syndrome** (Prenatal exposure to **Phenytoin**)
- Cleft lip, **C**ardiac defects**,** Long, thin fingers and toes; **C**onvex nails, **Meningomyelocele suggest → Fetal Valproate syndrome.**

Teratogenic effects of drugs	
Drug	**Effect**
Alcohol	Fetal alcohol syndrome
Isotretinoin	Facial, ear anomalies, congenital heart disease
Phenytoin	Hypoplastic nails, typical facies, IUGR
Diethylstilbestrol (DES)	Vaginal adenocarcinoma
Tetracycline	Enamel hypoplasia, discolored teeth
Lithium	Ebstein's anomaly
Warfarin	Facial dysmorphism and chondrodysplasia
Valproate/Carbamezapine	Mental retardation, neural tube defects
ACE inhibitors	Craniofacial abnormalities
Misoprostol	Moebius syndrome

5. **Ans. d. No need of treatment. Only home remedies.**

(Ref: IMNCI Protocols)

The keywords in this question hint towards the diagnosis of → Bronchiolitis

- MC agent implicated in causing Bronchiolitis = **Respiratory Syncytial Virus (RSV)**[Q] (> 50%); Others = parainfluenza, adenovirus, *Mycoplasma*, other viruses.
- **Typical age** = almost all children infected by **age < 2 years**[Q]; Most severe at age 1–2 months in winter months.
- Pathophysiology in a nutshell: Inflammation of the small airways → inflammatory obstruction: edema, mucus, and cellular debris → bilateral obstruction → air-trapping and overinflation.

Clinical Presentation

Signs and symptoms:

- Mild URI (often from household contact), decreased appetite and **fever**, irritability, paroxysmal wheezy cough, dyspnea, and **tachypnea**[Q]
- **Apnea** may be more prominent early in young infants.

Examination:

- Wheezing, increased work of breathing, fine crackles, prolonged expiratory phase.
- Lasts average of 12 days (worse in first 2–3 days)

Complications = bacterial superinfection, respiratory insufficiency and failure

Diagnosis:

- **Primarily clinical**[Q]
- Chest X-ray (not routine) = hyperinflation with patchy atelectasis (may mimic early pneumonia)
- Immunofluorescence of nasopharyngeal swab (not routine); PCR

Treatment:

- **Supportive care**[Q]; hospitalized, if respiratory distress.
- **No steroids**
- Ribavirin not routinely used; may prevent need for mechanical ventilation in severe cases

Prevention = Monoclonal Ab against RSV-F-protein (preferred: palivizumab) in high-risk patients only.

Extra Edge Info from Nelson 20/E:

- Additional risk factors = male gender, lack of breastfeeding and crowded conditions.
- Higher risk = infants with young mothers or mothers who smoked during pregnancy.
- Hypoxemia is a consequence of ventilation—perfusion mismatch early in the course. With severe obstructive disease and tiring of respiratory effort, hypercapnia can develop.

6. Ans. d. Chlamydia trachomatis

(Ref: Nelson Textbook of Pediatrics, 20/e p1495)

Conjunctivitis:

- Infants born to mothers with active, untreated chlamydial infection developing clinical conjunctivitis → Approx. 30–50%
- In Chlamydia infection, symptoms Most Commonly develop after **5–14 days** of delivery (Earlier in infants born after prolonged rupture of membranes).

- Conjunctiva → may be very **friable** and might **bleed** when stroked with a swab.
- Cases with Chlamydial conjunctivitis having **nasopharyngeal infection** = 50%.

Pneumonia:

- Characteristic presentation of C. trachomatis pneumonia of infancy is that the onset is often **insidious** and mostly occurs between → **1–3 months of age**, with **persistent cough, tachypnea**, and **absence of fever.**
- Auscultation findings = **rales**; [**wheezing** is uncommon].
- Absence of fever and wheezing are the distinguishing features of C. trachomatis pneumonia from Respiratory Syncytial Virus (RSV) pneumonia.
- Laboratory finding = presence of **peripheral eosinophilia (>400 cells/µL).**
- Most Consistent finding on chest radiograph = **hyperinflation** plus **minimal interstitial or alveolar infiltrates.**

Treatment:

- Recommended Rx for C. trachomatis conjunctivitis or pneumonia in infants is → erythromycin (50 mg/kg/day divided 4 times a day PO for 14 days) and azithromycin (20 mg/kg/day once daily PO for 3 days).

OBSTETRICS AND GYNECOLOGY

QUESTIONS

1. **A 32-year-old female came for routine PAP smear testing. The report came as carcinoma in situ. What is the next step?**
   a. Colposcopy and biopsy
   b. Conization
   c. Hysterectomy
   d. HPV DNA testing
2. **A Rh-negative mother, who has Indirect Coombs Test (ICT), negative was given Anti-D during 28-week of pregnancy. Which of the following is the ideal one?**
   a. Give another dose of Anti-D 72 hour postpartum depending on the baby blood group
   b. Give another dose of Anti-D 72 hour postpartum irrespective of baby blood group
   c. No need of additional dose since she is ICT negative
   d. All of the above
3. **Which of the following is a WHO guideline in second stage of labor?**
   a. Perform labor in lithotomy position
   b. Give warm compress to the perineum
   c. Manual support to perineum with deflexion of head
   d. Do a routine episiotomy
4. **Which of the following is the best parameter to assess in case of male infertility?**
   a. The number of sperm
   b. The morphology of sperms
   c. Motility of sperms
   d. Quantity of semen
5. **A mid aged women came to OPD with a twin pregnancy. She already had 2 first trimester abortion and she has a 3-year-old female child who was born at the end of ninth month of gestation. Which of the following is her accurate representation? G = gravid, P = para**
   a. G4P1 1+2+1   b. G5P1 2+0+1
   c. G4P1 0+1+2   d. G5P0 1+0+2

6. **From what cm of cervical dilatation is partogram plotted in regular intervals?**
   a. 4 cm b. 5 cm
   c. 6 cm d. 8 cm

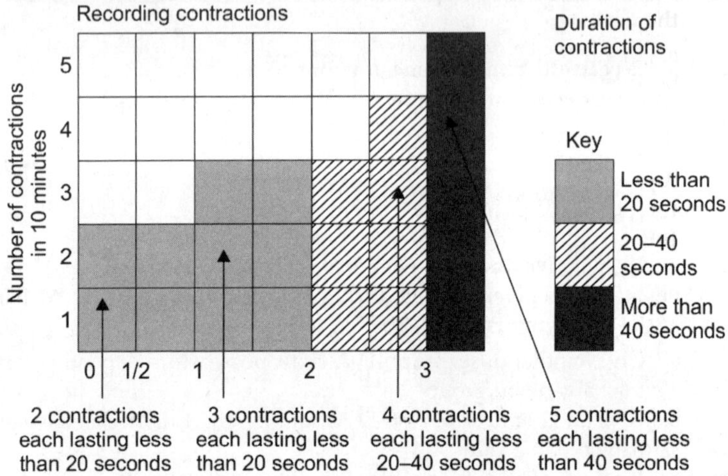

7. **A 25-year-old female worked up for primary infertility. On hysterosalpingography there was bilateral cornual block. Which is the next step in management?**
   a. Hydrotubation
   b. IVF
   c. Tuboplasty
   d. Hysteroscopy and laparoscopy guided surgery

8. **A 28-year-old female nearing her date has been admitted following regular contractions. The resident doctor did an examination and told the intern that the head is at +1 station. What does the exact position of head?**
   a. High up in the false pelvis
   b. Just above ischial spine
   c. Just below ischial spine
   d. At the perineum

9. **Which of the following fits into the criteria of severe variable deceleration, variations less than?**
   a. 70 beats per minute lasting for 60 seconds
   b. 80 beats per minute lasting for 60 seconds
   c. 90 beats per minute lasting for 60 seconds
   d. 100 beats per minute lasting for 60 seconds

10. A 59-year-old female with history of ovarian carcinoma in the mother achieved menopause with smooth transition. And she is on hormone replacement therapy. She developed abdominal pain and the right adnexal mass was palpable, non tender. On routine examination she has a 3 × 3 cm smooth cyst in her ovary. Which is the next step?

a. Do CA-125 levels, if normal advise regular checkup
b. Confirm USG findings by ordering CT scan
c. Do an exploratory laparoscopy to visualize the nature of cyst
d. Reassure and advice regular follow up once in 6 months

11. A pregnant lady was admitted for pregnancy induced hypertension for monitoring and bed rest. In supine position which of the following is a complication of the below representation?

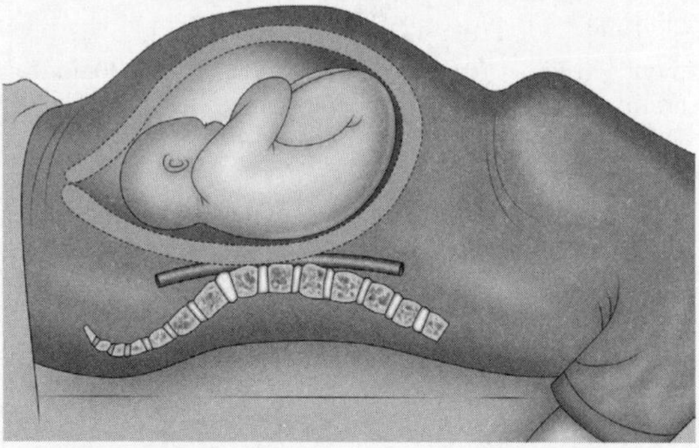

a. Abdominal aorta syndrome
b. Supine vena cava syndrome
c. Superior vena cava syndrome
d. Ascending aorta syndrome

12. A 23-year-old female came with complaints of 4 months amenorrhea. The FSH and LH were elevated above the normal value. Thyroid function test were normal. Which is the next step in management?

a. Give progesterone and stop after 10 days for withdrawal bleeding
b. Check USG for polycystic ovaries
c. Estimate serum estradiol values
d. Do a urine pregnancy test

13. Ureteric injury is most commonly associated with which of the following?

a. Anterior colporrhaphy
b. Vaginal hysterectomy
c. Wertheim hysterectomy
d. Abdominal hysterectomy

EXPLANATIONS

1. Ans. a. Colposcopy and biopsy *(Ref: ASCCP Guidelines)*

Below are the standard guidelines for operation in PAP smear reporting:

Test Results	What to Do Next
Normal Pap and Negative HPV	Rescreen in 5 years.
Normal Pap and Positive HPV	Repeat co-test in one year or do HPV DNA typing now
ASCUS Pap, No HPV Test	Repeat cytology in one year or do HPV test now
ASCUS Pap and Negative HPV LSIL Pap and Negative HPV	Repeat Pap and co-test at interval as per ASCCP guidelines.
ASCUS Pap and Positive HPV LSIL Pap and Positive or unknown HPV ASC-H Pap HSIL Pap	Colposcopy and biopsy and/or referral to gynecologist.

Extra Edge: Some surgical procedures:

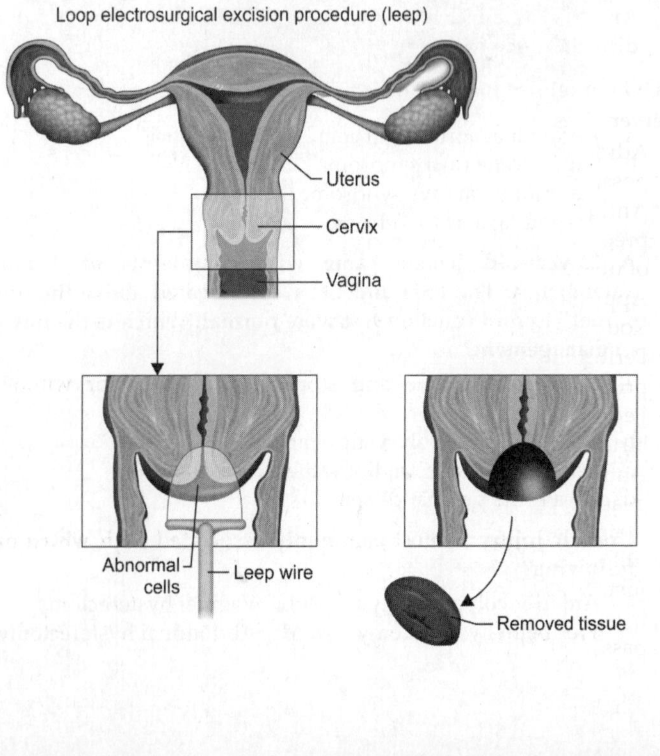

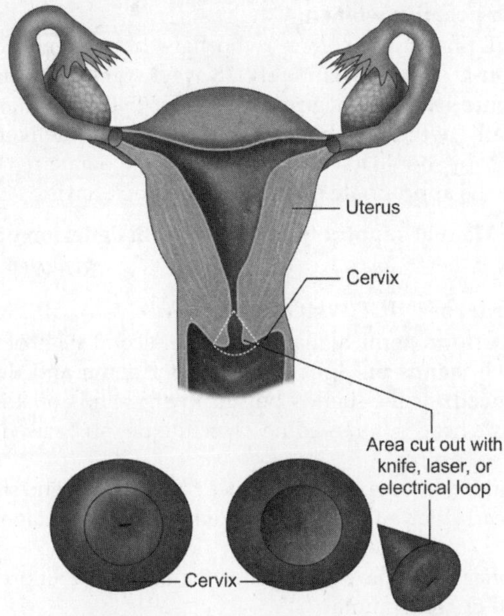

2. **Ans. a. Give another dose of Anti-D 72 hours postpartum depending on the baby blood group** *(Ref: RCOG Guidelines)*

RCOG guidelines for Anti-D prophylaxis in various situations
Interventions and Practices considered:

- Administration of anti-D immunoglobulin (anti-D Ig) as soon as possible after potentially sensitizing events.
- Anti-D Ig prophylaxis (following an ectopic pregnancy, molar pregnancy, therapeutic termination of pregnancy and in some cases of uterine bleeding).
- Appropriate testing for fetomaternal hemorrhage (FMH).
- Routine antenatal prophylaxis with anti-D Ig (RAADP).
- Performing 28-weeks sample for blood group and antibody screen prior to first routine prophylactic anti-D Ig injection.
- Performing ABO and rhesus (Rh) D typing on cord blood following birth.
- Anti-D Ig prophylaxis in the event of a D positive child or intrauterine death.
- Maintenance of auditable records of issue and administration to allow full traceability of anti-D Ig.
- Investigation performed when anti-D is detected in a blood sample from a pregnant woman to establish whether this is immune or passive.

Anti-D in Rh-negative women:

- All Rh (D) negative women (who have not actively formed their own Anti-D) at **approximately 28 weeks gestation** and again at approximately 34 weeks gestation - CSL 625 IU (125 mcg).
- Postnatally, within 72 hours. All women who deliver an Rh (D) positive baby should have quantification of fetomaternal hemorrhage to guide the appropriate dose of anti-D prophylaxis.

3. **Ans. c. Manual support to perineum with deflexion of head**

(Ref: WHO Guidelines)

Second stage labor (NICE/WHO guidelines)

- Do not perform perineal massage in the second stage of labor.
- Either the **'hands on' (guarding the perineum and deflexing the baby's head)** or the 'hands poised' (with hands off the perineum and baby's head but in readiness) technique can be used to facilitate spontaneous birth.
- Do not offer lidocaine spray to reduce pain in the second stage of labor.
- Do not carry out a routine episiotomy during spontaneous vaginal birth.
- Do not offer episiotomy routinely at vaginal birth after previous third- or fourth-degree trauma.

A useful table on stages of labor:

Stage	First Stage			Second Stage	Third Stage	Fourth Stage
Overall Function	Cervix	Thins and Opens		Pushing and Birth	Birth of Placenta	Bonding, Resting, Nursing
Phase	Early Labor	Active Labor	Transition			
Contractions	5–20 min. apart Last 30–60 sec.	3–5 min. apart Last 60 sec.	2–3 min. apart Last 60–90 sec. May have double peaks or no rests in between	May space out to 5 min. apart. Last 60 sec.	Stimulated by nursing Usually 3–5 min. apart	The more children you have, the more you may experience afterbirth pains
Cervix	0–6 cm dilation	6–8 cm dilation	8–10 cm dilation	10 cm dilation		
Mental/ Emotional changes	Excited Nervous Talkative	Inward Focused Cannot talk	Frustrated Dependent Crying "I can't do it!"!	Recharged, excited, alert and aware	Relieved Happy Tired	Love for baby, Fatigue

Contd...

Contd...

Stage	First Stage			Second Stage	Third Stage	Fourth Stage
Length	6–12+ hours	3–5 hours	30 min. (–)2+ hours	20 min. –4+ hours	5 min. – 1 hour	First 24 hours

4. **Ans. b. The morphology of sperms**

(Ref: WHO Manual for the Examination & Processing of Human Semen 5/e, 2010)

Semen:

Constituents:

- Sperms from the testis—10%
- Seminal vesicle-alkaline—70%
- Prostate—acidic—20%
- Final pH—alkaline

Semen analysis:

- Volume > 1.5 mL
- Sperm concentration > 15 million/mL
- Motility > 40%
- Progressive motility > 32%
- Morphology > 4% normal forms
- Pus cells should be absent
- pH—alkaline (8)
- Fructose—150–600 mg %
- Leukocyte < 1 million/mL
- Vitality > 75% living
- Liquefies in 20–30 minutes

The most important parameter is Sperm morphology.

"**Morphology of spermatozoa.** Morphology is also a very important parameter of the quality of spermatozoa. To analyze their morphology, sperm cells undergo a specialized screening, using individualized observation under a light microscope. In a fertile sample, spermatozoa with a normal morphology should exceed **5%**".

5. **Ans. c. G4P1 0+1+2** *(Ref: OBG Terminology and Definitions)*

The nomenclature for this question is based on a system called GTPAL system.

TPAL terminology= A system used to describe obstetrical history.

- **T** = Term births
- **P** = Preterm births (prior to 37 weeks gestation)
- **A** = Abortions
- **L** = Living children

The GPA terminology is combined with TPAL terminology → GTPAL terminology.

So, Patient describe in the question will be represented as (live is included as Para 1)

G4 P1 (0+1+2)

6. **Ans. a. 4 cm** *(Ref: WHO)*

Partograph:

- The partograph is a graphic record of the progress of labor and relevant details of the mother and fetus.
- The WHO partograph begins only in the active phase of labour, when the cervix is 4 cm or more dilated.

Observations to be made:

- **Maternal well-being:** record pulse rate every 30 minutes, blood pressure and temperature 4-hourly, urine output and dipstick testing for protein, ketones (if available) and glucose after voiding, and record all fluids and drugs administered. If the findings become abnormal, increased frequency of observation and testing will be required, and intervention may be implemented.
- **Fetal well-being:** record fetal heart rate for 1 minute every 15–30 minutes after a contraction in the first stage, and every 5 minutes in the second stage. If abnormalities are noted, urgent delivery can be considered.
- **Liquor:** clear, meconium stained (thick or thin), bloody or absent. Thick meconium suggests fetal distress, and closer monitoring of the fetus is indicated. Check every 30 minutes.
- **Moulding:**
  - 0 = bones are separated and sutures can be easily felt;
  - + 1 = bones are just touching each other;
  - + 2 = bones are overlapping but can be reduced;
  - + 3 = bones are severely overlapping and irreducible.
- Cervical dilatation: assess at each VE and mark with a cross ×. Begin at 4 cm.
- Alert line: starting at 4 cm of cervical dilatation, up to the point of expected full dilatation at the rate of 1 cm per hour.
- Action line: parallel and 4 hours to the right of the alert line.
- Descent assessed by abdominal palpation: this refers to the part of the head (which is divided into five parts) palpable above the symphysis pubis; recorded as a circle (O) at every vaginal examination. At 0/5, the sinciput (S) is at the level of the symphysis pubis.

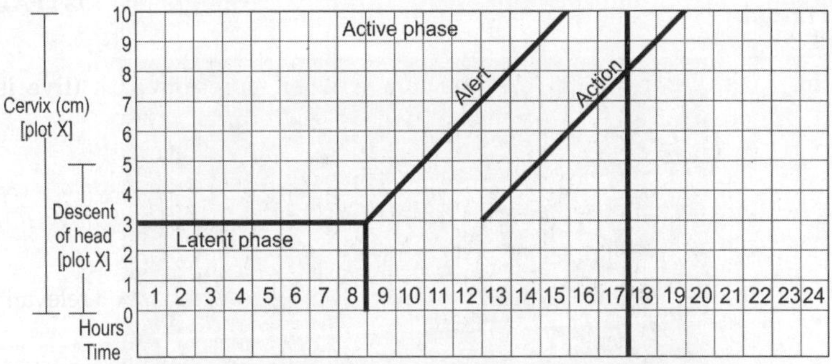

7. **Ans. d. Hysteroscopy and laparoscopy guided surgery**

(Ref: ACOG Guidelines)

This is a practical question and a bit tricky.

Bilateral tubal block in hysterosalpingography, one should not jump into the diagnosis that it's pathological.

- One of the most common cause of bilateral tubal block is—can be due to spasm of the sphincters present in the corneal region. So the first step is to confirm whether the block is due to spasm (as a result of pain) or really pathological.
- To differentiate this, one must do a diagnostic laparoscopy, so answer is D.

Hysteroscopy (diagnostic as well as therapeutic)

- Remove **adhesions** that may occur because of infection or from past surgery.
- Diagnose the cause of repeated **miscarriage** when a woman has more than two miscarriages in a row.
- Locate an **intrauterine device.**
- Perform **sterilization**, in which the hysteroscope is used to place small implants into a woman's **fallopian tubes** as a permanent form of birth control.

Images of Hysterosalpingography:

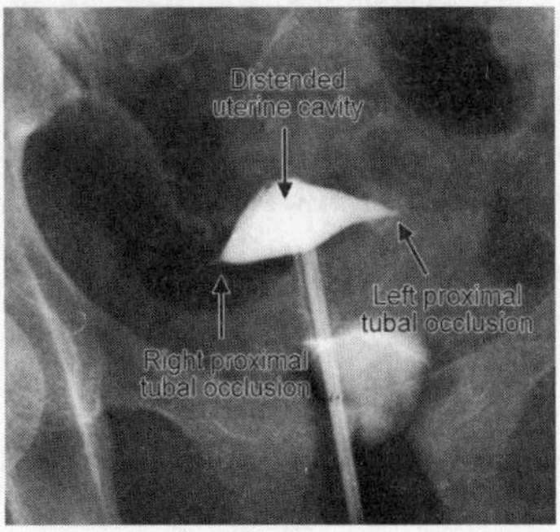

Fibroid:

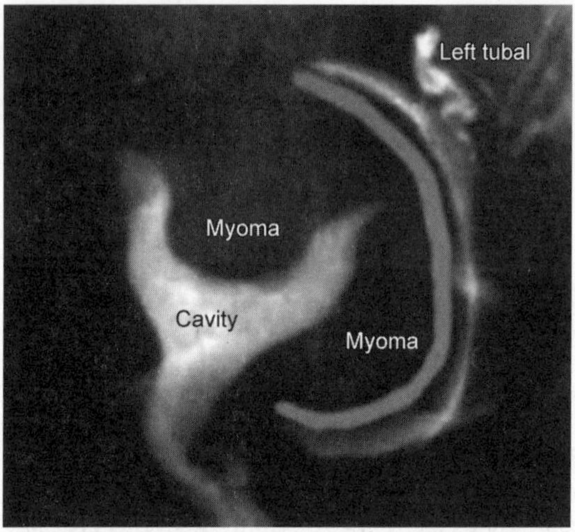

Bicornuate uterus:

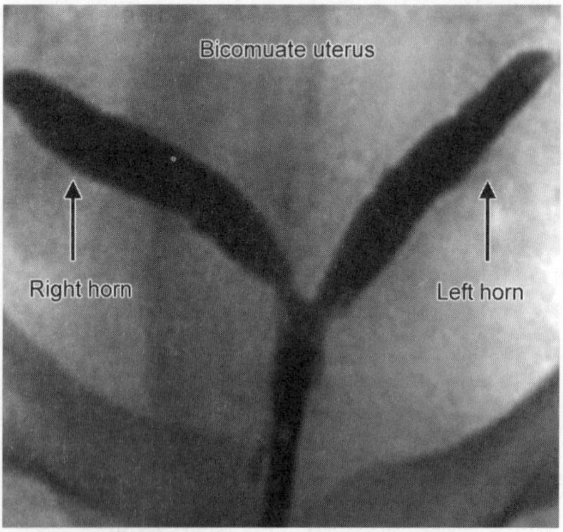

8. **Ans. c. Just below ischial spine**

(Ref: Clinical Practice Guidelines Obstetrics, p213)

Station of head:

Fetal station describes how far down baby's head has descended into your pelvis.

Score	Position
5 to 0	The "presenting" or most palpable (able to feel) part of the baby is above the woman's ischial spines. Sometimes a doctor can't feel the presenting part. This station is known as the "floating."
Zero station	The baby's head is known to be "engaged," or aligned with the ischial spines.
0 to +5	Positive numbers are used when a baby has descended beyond the ischial spines. During birth a baby is at the +4 to +5 station.

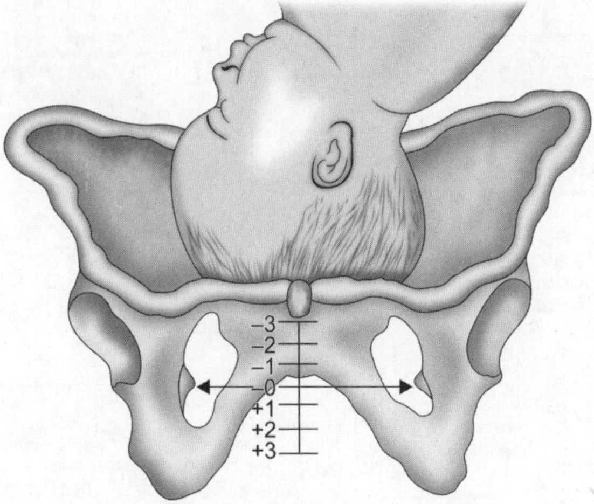

9. **Ans. a. 70 beats per minute lasting for 60 seconds**
(Ref: NICHD Guidelines)

This question is based on the classification of variable decelerations.

Classification of variable decelerations:

- Mild: > 80 bpm irrespective of duration or < 30 seconds irrespective of depth or 70 to 80 bpm lasting for 60 seconds
- Moderate: > 70 bpm lasting for 30–60 seconds or 70–80 bpm lasting for ≥ 60 seconds
- Severe: < 70 bpm lasting at least 60 seconds

10. **Ans. a. Do CA-125 levels, if normal advise regular checkup**
(Ref: RCOG Guidelines)

This question is again based on the recent guidelines for management of postmenopausal ovarian cysts by RCOG.

Abbreviations
BSO bilateral salingo-oophorectomy
CT computed tomography
MDT multidisciplinary team
RMI risk of malignancy index
TAH total abdominal hysterectomy
TAS transabdominal scanning
TVS transvaginal scanning

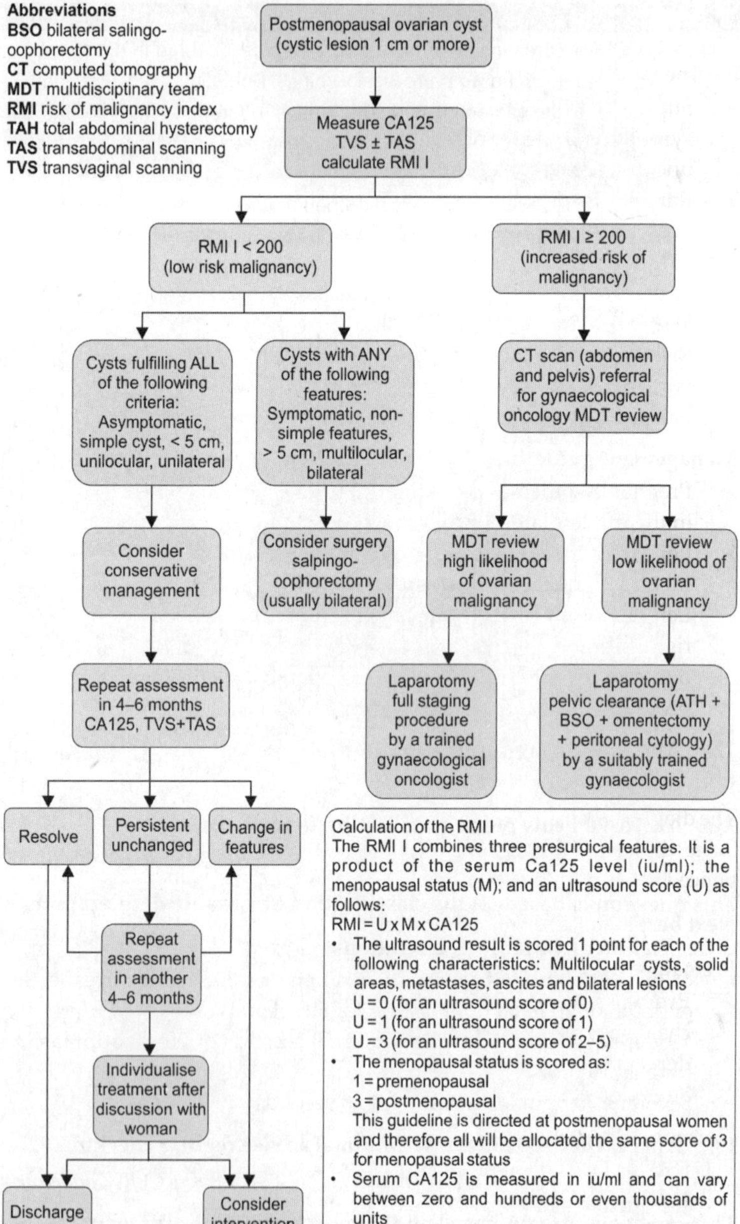

Calculation of the RMI I

The RMI I combines three presurgical features. It is a product of the serum Ca125 level (iu/ml); the menopausal status (M); and an ultrasound score (U) as follows:

RMI = U x M x CA125

- The ultrasound result is scored 1 point for each of the following characteristics: Multilocular cysts, solid areas, metastases, ascites and bilateral lesions
  U = 0 (for an ultrasound score of 0)
  U = 1 (for an ultrasound score of 1)
  U = 3 (for an ultrasound score of 2–5)
- The menopausal status is scored as:
  1 = premenopausal
  3 = postmenopausal
  This guideline is directed at postmenopausal women and therefore all will be allocated the same score of 3 for menopausal status
- Serum CA125 is measured in iu/ml and can vary between zero and hundreds or even thousands of units

11. **Ans. b. Supine vena cava syndrome**

(Ref: Williams Obstetrics, p1369)

Supine vena cava/ Supine hypotensive syndrome:

- Supine hypotensive syndrome is characterized by severe supine symptoms and hypotension in late pregnancy, which compel the unconstrained subject to change position.
- Rarely, it may manifest even from the fifth month of pregnancy or postpartum, as well as in the pelvic tilt or sitting positions.
- 15% of women at term can demonstrate supine hypotensive syndrome of pregnancy, defined as a decrease in systolic blood pressure of at least 15–30 mm Hg.
- Risk factors are more common with multiple pregnancies and obese parturients. In addition, the syndrome is exacerbated by neuraxial blocks due to the cofounding sympathectomy.

Management guidelines:

- Pregnant women at more than 20 weeks gestation should be placed in the full left lateral position when recumbent.
- Left lateral position is preferred, but other options include left lateral tilt and manual displacement of the gravid uterus.
- Left lateral tilt to 15°–30° is achieved by placing a wedge under the right hip and is used in practice for labor and delivery as well as nonobstetric surgery in pregnant patients undergoing anesthesia to prevent supine hypotensive syndrome.

12. **Ans. c. Estimate serum estradiol values**

(Ref: Clinical Reproductive Medicine, William Hurd, p288)

The diagnosis here is Premature ovarian failure, dd of which is pregnancy. Since the levels of LH and FSH are high, it cannot be pregnancy and hence UPT is not advised here. !!!

Next best step is Serum estradiol:

Premature ovarian failure:

- Premature ovarian failure (POF) is a primary ovarian defect characterized by absent menarche (primary amenorrhea) or premature depletion of ovarian follicles before the age of 40 years (secondary amenorrhea).

Hormonal levels:

- FSH, LH will be high
- Low serum estradiol levels
- High levels of serum prolactin.

Other tests:

- Karyotype
- FMR1 gene testing

13. Ans. c. Wertheim hysterectomy

(Ref: Textbook of Obstetrics, Sudha Salhan, p17)

- Ureteric injury has an incidence of 0.2–1.0% during any abdominal or pelvic surgery.
- The most high risk is for Wertheim followed by adenexectomy.

Sites of injury:

The most notable sites of ureteric injury are:

- At the pelvic brim as the infundibulopelvic ligament is being divided (in 30 percent of cases).
- The ovarian fossa during resection of ovaries or ovarian remnants (in 19 percent of cases).
- Lateral to the cervix during division of the uterine artery, the uterosacral ligament and the cardinal ligament (in 51 percent of cases).
- The left ureter is more commonly damaged in the pelvis than the right, because the position of the right ureter is almost always constant and crosses the external iliac artery, whereas the left lies closer to the midline and crosses the common iliac artery.

DERMATOLOGY

QUESTIONS

1. **The following patient came with history of hair loss. There were no complaints of erythema, scarring and scratching. Diagnosis is:**

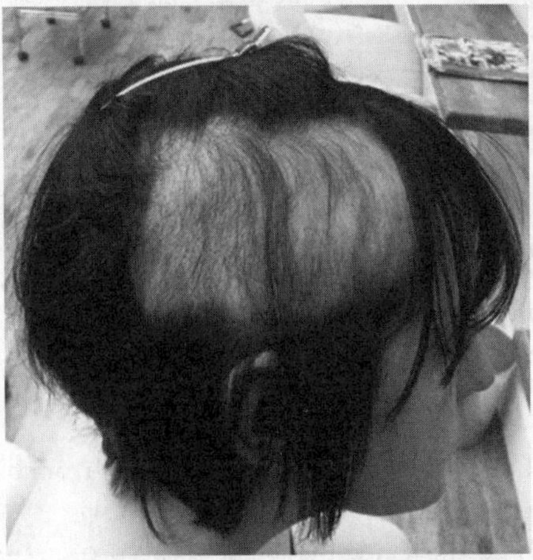

(See Color Plate 11)

a. Trichotillomania
b. Alopecia areata
c. Telogen effluvium
d. Tinea infection

2. **A 12-year-old gives history of red lesions with itching and discharges on flexure aspect of elbow. Diagnosis is:**

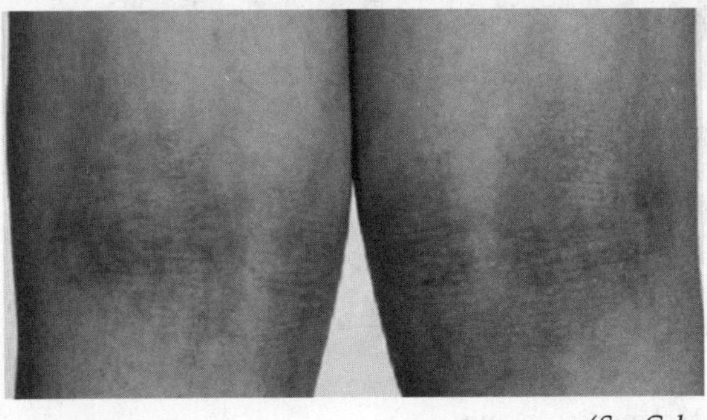

(See Color Plate 11)

a. Psoriasis
b. Atopic dermatitis
c. Pemphigus vulgaris
d. Post-traumatic pigmentation

3. **The below patient presented with itching and mild discharge and hair loss. Which of the following is useful for diagnosis?**

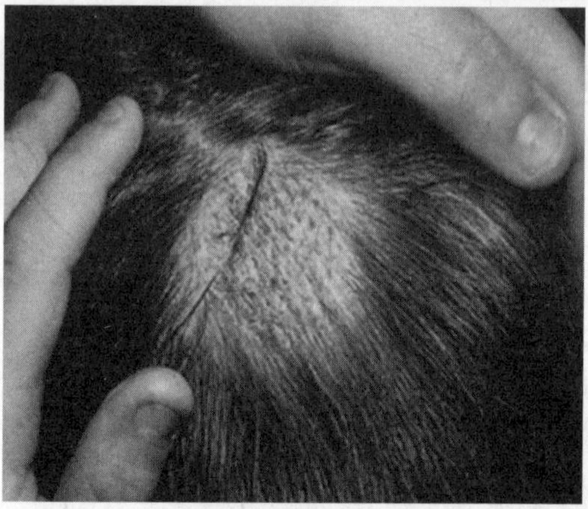

(See Color Plate 12)

a. Gram stain
b. Slit skin smear
c. KOH mount
d. Tzanck smear

4. **Identify the below condition which is present from birth:**

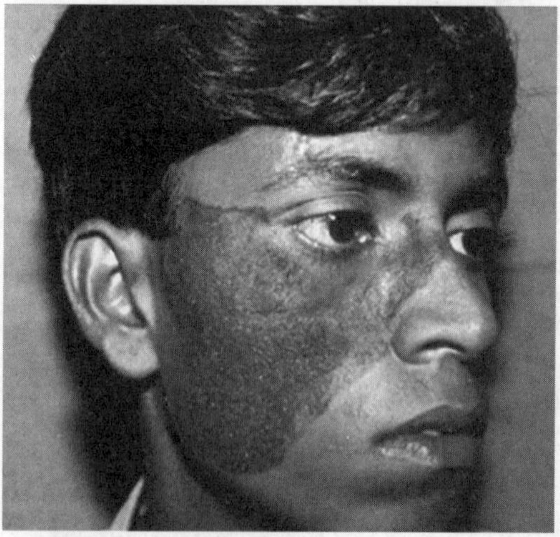

(See Color Plate 12)

a. Epidermal verrucous nevus
b. Melanoacanthoma
c. Congenital nevus
d. Malignant melanoma

EXPLANATIONS

1. **Ans. a. Trichotillomania**

(Ref: Rook's Textbook of Dermatology, 9/e, p86.17-86.1)

Differential points:

- Trichotillomania is not necessarily associated with erythema/some cases do have erythema. But presence of erythema does not rule out the diagnosis
- Alopecia areata will be more regular in shape and density

Alopecia: Look at the more regular patterned hair loss

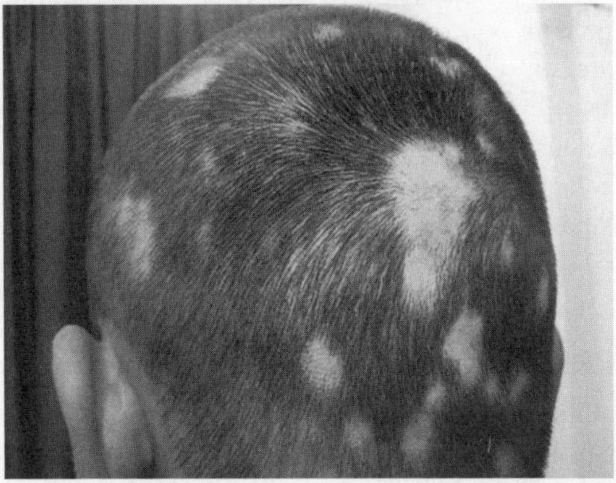

Alopecia – Histopathology – Swarm of bees appearance (NBE question), the lymphocytes surrounding the hair follicles.

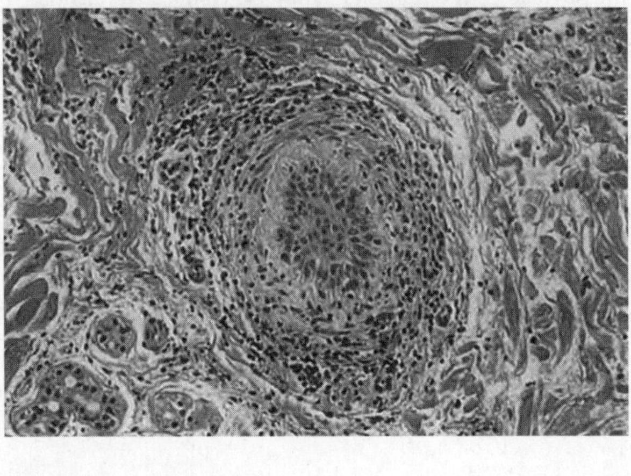

Trichotillomania

- Trichotillomania is a behavioral disorder characterized by compulsive hair-pulling
- It presents as a pattern of hair loss, often bizarre, with no clear biological or overt traumatic explanation.
- Hair is plucked most frequently from one frontoparietal region.
- This results in a patch of hair loss, often in a bizarre or angular pattern, in which the hairs are twisted and broken at various distances from the clinically normal scalp.

2. **Ans. b. Atopic dermatitis**

(Ref: Fitzpatrick's Dermatology in General Medicine, 8/e, p165)

Atopic dermatitis is a chronic or chronically relapsing disorder with major features of:

- Pruritus
- Eczematous dermatitis (acute, subacute, or chronic) with typical morphology and age-specific patterns
- Facial and extensor involvement in infancy, and
- Flexural eczema/lichenification in children and adults.

3. **Ans. c. KOH mount**

(Ref: Fitzpatrick's Dermatology in General Medicine, 8/e, p2284-5)

The clinical diagnosis here is Tinea capitis:

- Infection of hair by dermatophytes follows 3 main patterns—ectothrix, endothrix and favus.
- Using KOH examination, in ectothrix infections, only the arthroconidia on the surface of the hair shaft may be visualized, although hyphae are also present within the hair shaft. The cuticle is destroyed. There may be circumscribed erythematous scaly patches of nonscarring alopecia with breakage of hairs: "gray patch" type. On Wood's lamp examination, a yellow-green fluorescence may be detected, depending on the causative organism.
- In endothrix infections, arthroconidia and hyphae remain within the hair shaft and leave the cortex and cuticle intact. This pattern of tinea capitis is associated with the appearance of "black dots" which represent broken hairs at the surface of the scalp.
- Favus is characterized by longitudinally arranged hyphae and air spaces within the hair shaft. Arthroconidia are not usually noted in infected hairs.

KOH mount:

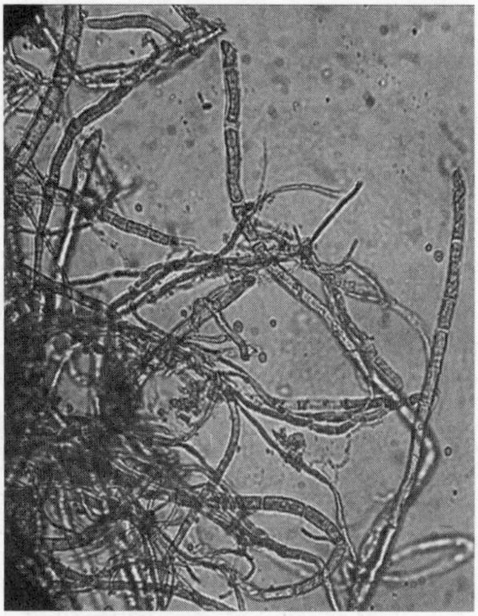

Other option for diagnosis: (Wood's lamp)

- Tinea capitis—areas of scale and baldness due to fungal infection.
- Microsporum species fluoresce blue-green (M. canis, M. audouinii, M. ferrugineum, M. distortum)
- Trichophyton schoenleinii fluoresces dull blue.
- Fungal infection due to other organisms does not fluoresce.

Wood's lamp:

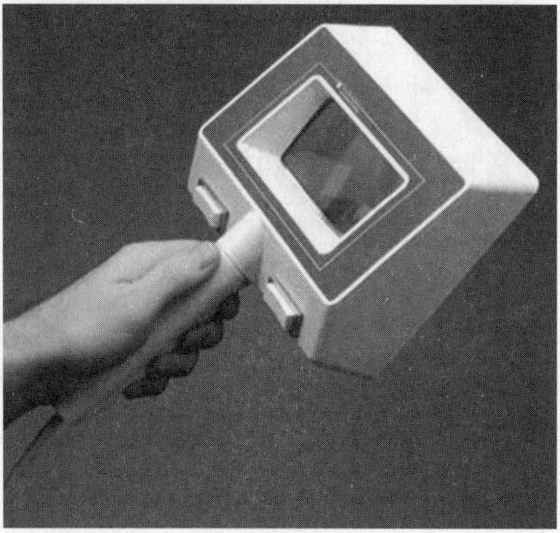

4. **Ans. c. Congenital nevus**

Congenital nevus:

- Congenital melanocytic nevus present at birth or shortly thereafter.
- Synonyms: Garment nevus, giant pigmented nevus.
- Lesions may be small or cover a substantial portion of the body surface
- Nevi are generally darker than the surrounding skin, have a rugose or smooth elevated surface and may demonstrate long, darker, thicker hairs.
- Large lesions have a significant risk of melanoma development.
- Cranial or midline lesions and large congenital nevomelanocytic nevus lesions with satellite lesions have an increased risk of leptomeningeal involvement.
- Often exhibit extensive nevomelanocytic infiltration of the dermis with potential involvement of the underlying adipose and muscular tissue.

Histopathology:

Proliferative nodules:

- Dermal nodules of large epithelioid or spindled melanocytes that merge with surrounding nevus cells.
- Often prominent nucleoli, cellular areas, focal hemorrhage and ulceration, but no necrosis, no destructive growth, minimal inflammation and 0-4 mitotic figures/10 HPF.

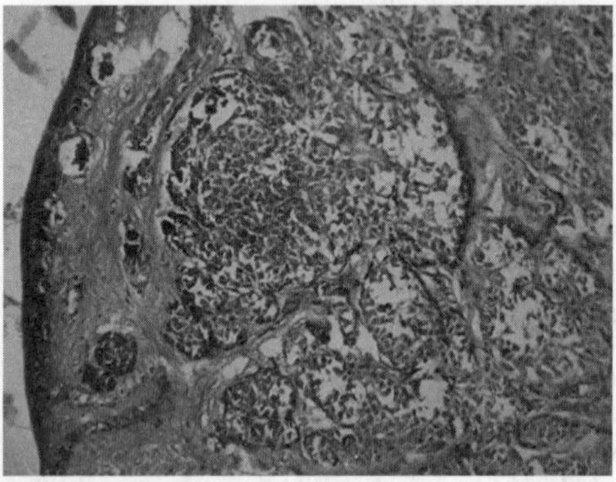

ANESTHESIA

QUESTION

1. **All are true about the procedure done by this needle *except*:**

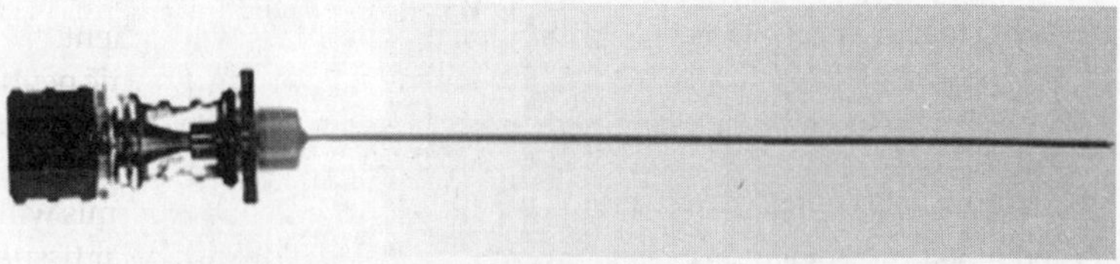

   a. Breath-holding is not necessary
   b. Coagulopathy is not an absolute contraindication
   c. The bevel should face upwards while inserting the needle
   d. To be done in lateral recumbent position

EXPLANATION

1. **Ans. b. Coagulopathy is not an absolute contraindication**

(Ref: Morgan, Anesthesia 5/e, p948)

Absolute contraindications to spinal anesthesia:
❍ Patient refusal
❍ Sepsis at the site of injection
❍ Hypovolemia
❍ Coagulopathy
❍ Indeterminate neurologic disease
❍ Increased intracranial pressure

Relative contraindications:
❍ Infection distinct from the site of injection
❍ Unknown duration of surgery

Miller anesthesia textbook says it is relative contraindication, even then the best one to choose will be option b.

- Lumbar puncture – is usually done in lateral recumbent position.
- The sitting position is utilized for low lumbar or sacral anesthesia and in instances when the patient is obese and there is difficulty in finding the midline in the lateral position.
- When performing a saddle block, the patient should remain in the sitting position for at least 5 minutes after a hyperbaric spinal anesthetic is placed to allow the spine to settle into that region.
- Bevel face upwards towards ceiling in lateral decubitus and towards flank in sitting position parallel to the muscle fibre.
- Breath-holding is not necessary to do lumbar puncture.

RADIOLOGY

QUESTIONS

1. **Following is not a finding in the chest X-ray given below:**

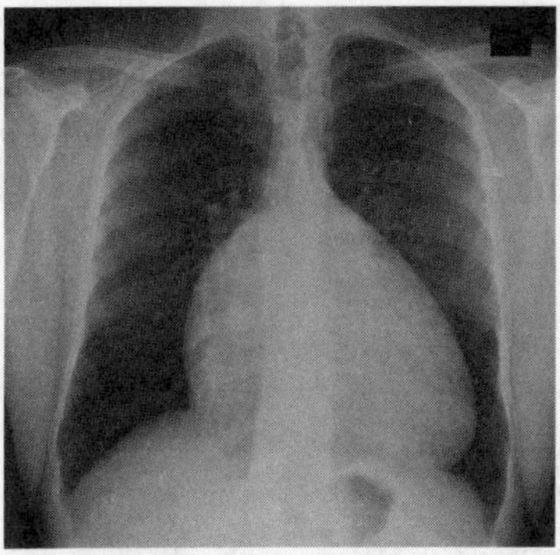

a. Narrow vascular pedicle
b. Right atrial enlargement
c. Decreased pulmonary blood flow
d. Pulmonary venous hypertension

2. **The following is a THYROID SCAN. The most probable diagnosis can be:**

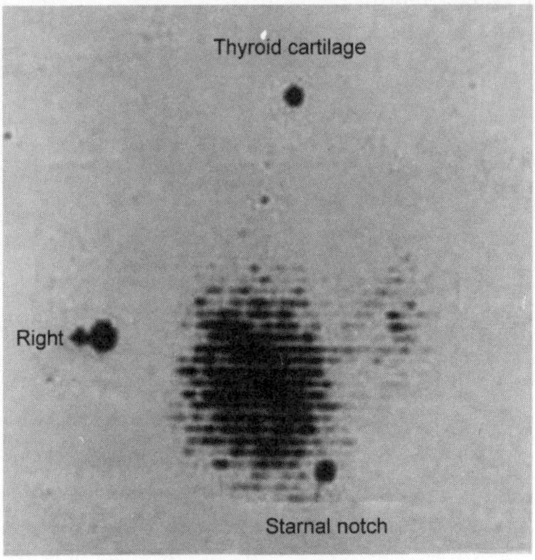

a. Papillary Ca thyroid
b. Lateral aberrant thyroid
c. Hypersecreting adenoma
d. Grave's disease

3. **A 50-year-old banker underwent routine USG. USG showed complex cyst in kidney with an exophytic mass. CT scan is shown below. Diagnosis is:**

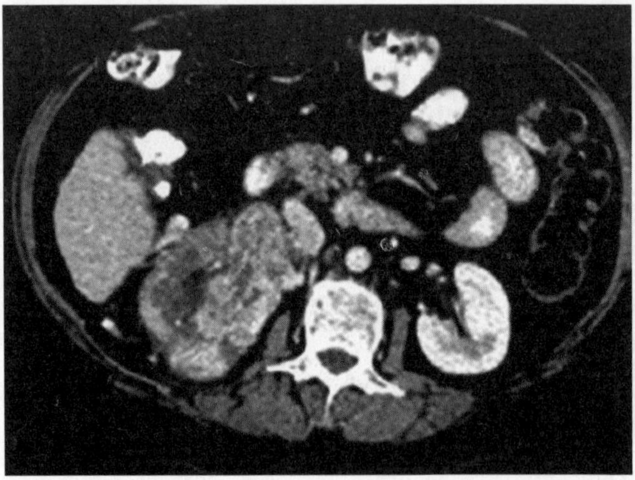

a. Renal angiomyolipoma
b. Parapelvic cyst
c. Renal cell carcinoma
d. Renal cyst

EXPLANATIONS

1. Ans. d. Pulmonary venous hypertension

(Ref: Chest X-ray Made Easy, Jonathan Corne, p108)

To solve the above question, we need to start with a normal chest X-ray.

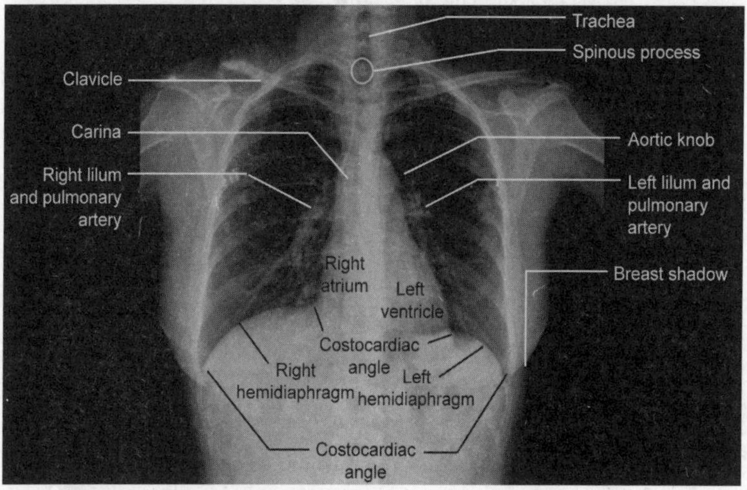

The CXR given shows the following:

- Cardiomegaly
- Narrow vascular pedicles
- Hyperlucent lung fields → suggestive of decreased pulmonary flow
- No pulmonary hypertension in this case.

Hence the possible diagnosis based on the given findings can be pulmonary hypertension: Pulmonary venous hypertension, if present, will show prominant hilar vessels, plethoric lung fields.

EXTRA EDGE: One more differential diagnosis can be seen—Severe valvular regurgitation involving right side of heart.

2. Ans. c. Hypersecreting adenoma.

(Ref: Essentials of Nuclear Medicine Imaging, Fred A Milter p605; The History of Radiology, Adrian MK Thomas p186)

Thyroid scan (IMPORTANT FACTS)
❍ Functional scan
❍ Patient preparation – NPO for 4 hours prior to exam
❍ Radiopharmaceutical agent of choice – Tc-99m pertechnetate

Contd...

Contd...

❍ Dose and route of administration 3–5 mCi IV
❍ Time of imaging – 20 minutes after dose
❍ Equipment: ❑ Gamma camera ❑ Pinhole collimator ❑ 20% energy window centered at 140 KeV[Q]
❍ Procedure: ❑ Obtain anterior, LAO, and RAO views ❑ Mark chin, suprasternal notch, palpable nodules, and surgical scars

Findings

- Suppressed UPTAKE in left lobe and increased UPTAKE in right lobe
- **Diagnosis –Toxic nodule which is hyperfunctioning and suppressing the uptake in left lobe of thyroid.**

EXTRA EDGE

- Malignancy does not uptake any dye (cold spots)
- The Duke 3-tiered system guidelines are used for thyroid nodules now

The following is a summary of the findings:

- The 3-tiered system reduces FNA rate for incidental thyroid nodules by 34–46%
- The 3-tiered system captures the same proportion of thyroid cancers compared to a 1 cm size cut off
- Incidental thyroid cancers missed by the 3-tiered system represent 1% of all thyroid cancers having surgery and are small papillary cancers that are lower in stage
- The 3-tiered system results in a net 54% reduction in ITN reported in the impression section of the report.

3. **Ans. c. Renal cell carcinoma**
   - A 50-year-old male with a complex renal cyst found out as an incidental finding
   - The CT picture shows an exophytic enhancing mass arising from the right kidney inferior pole and extending towards midline with disruption of perinephric fat points in favor of renal cell carcinoma.

Other options – negative findings

- Other options like renal cyst and parapelvic cyst are simple cysts and so they are ruled out, as USG says complex cyst.

- Angiomyolipoma can be the next best option if RCC was not mentioned as both are seen as incidental findings (more in case of AML) but:
  - AML is more common in females.
  - RCC is more common in 40–50 years in males and also incidentally diagnosed due to recent increase in the use of imaging.
  - RCC and AML both can present as exophytic mass, but RCC has cystic component too, whereas AML is not associated with cysts and contains more amount of fat and vascular structures, thus leaving us with the option of RCC.

PSYCHIATRY

QUESTIONS

1. **Mutism and akinesis in a person in awake state is a feature of:**
   a. Oneiroid state
   b. Stupor
   c. Twilight state
   d. Delirium

2. **Which of the following mood stabilizer has anti-suicidal role?**
   a. Lithium
   b. Carbamazepine
   c. Valproate
   d. Lamotrigine

3. **A 20-year-old female has thoughts of cutting her fingers, she plans and imagines doing it but never actually does it. She says that she is not having any guilt of having such thought. And also says the thoughts are distressing her and she is unable to control them. The thoughts vanish either by ending with a seizure or automatically subsides on its own. Which of the following is the cause?**
   a. Obsession
   b. Thought insertion
   c. Forced thinking
   d. Crowding of thoughts

4. **A patient suffering from a known case of psychotic disorder on anitpsychotics and antihypertensives on treatment. He suddenly developed tachycardia and chest tightness. On evaluation he had metabolic acidosis. ECG showed—widened QRS complex and prolonged QT interval. Which of the following drug is responsible for this?**
   a. Amlodipine
   b. Amitriptyline
   c. Enalapril
   d. Chlorthalidone

EXPLANATIONS

1. Ans. b. Stupor *(Ref: A Short Textbook of Psychiatry. Ahuja. 7/e, p239)*

This is a repeat question. And it's in Dr. Bhatia Discussion slides..!!

Stupor:

- There is severe reduction of relational function, that is speech and action occurs i.e. akinetic mutism, patient unable to initiate action and speech but appears awake and alert.
- A syndrome called "Locked In Syndrome" occur when there is involvement of motor pathways in ventral pons characterized by quadriplegia, anarthria (inability to articulate remembered words as a result of a brain lesion) with retained consciousness and vertical eye movement.

Oneiroid state:

- It is also called dreamlike state and is defined by the fantastic psychological suffering. It is characterized by ambivalent, contradictory speech, criminal action, senses global, changing, catastrophe, and celebration simultaneously.
- Oneiroid is frequently met with vivid hallucination and illusion which are perceived not as a real fact in the world but as a presentation, like a movie (psuedohallucination).

Twilight state:

- Twilight states: They are present in typical epileptic paroxysm.
- Psychosis is characterized by sudden onset, very short duration and abrupt end with total amnesia for the total period of disorder of consciousness.
- Symptoms may be different for different patients. But some common factors are present.
- Perception of the surrounding is partial; patient snatches out from the surrounding irritated facts and reacts at them unpredictably.

Delirium: This is acute psychosis with obscured consciousness, and is accompanied by illusion, hallucination scenario, disturbances of orientation of time, place (but not self-orientation or personality) and abrupt psychomotor excitement.

Amentia: This is a rough obscured consciousness with incoherent thought, complete unavailability for contact, isolated deception of perception and signs of sudden physical exhaustion.

2. **Ans. a. Lithium** *(Ref: A Short Textbook of Psychiatry. Ahuja. 7/e, p203)*

Lithium:

- Lithium is used as a psychiatric treatment against the recurrence of mania and as a treatment, and prophylaxis for depressive disorders.
- Lithium may have some antidepressant effects but these are less than those of less-toxic agents such as tricyclics. Lithium has also been claimed to be of use in reduction of premenstrual tension.
- Lithium-enhanced use of high dose tricyclics is a treatment alternative for depressive illness where the use of high dose tricyclics alone has failed to have a therapeutic effect.
- Lithium is DOC for acute mania, bipolar depression as well as augmenting agent in treatment resistant depression along with anti-depressants.
- Lithium has unique action that it is very useful for maintenance of bipolar 1 disorder or mania.
- Lithium reduces the incidence of suicide in bipolar 1 disorder 6 to 7 folds, this anti-suicidal property is also seen in Clozapine [2nd generation-anti-psychotic agent].
- MC Side effect of Lithium is–Neurological, i.e. tremors.

3. **Ans. c. Forced thinking** *(Ref: Lishman's Organic Psychiatry 4/e, p557)*

This is a classical case of forced thinking. The thoughts here is the aura

- Forced thinking (FT) is a rare epileptic phenomenon which is usually seen in patients with frontal lobe epilepsy.
- FT is a rare type of aura that refers to recurrent intrusive thoughts, ideas, or crowding of thoughts.
- FT is generally considered as a type of psychic auras. Other types of psychic auras comprise complex visual or auditory hallucination or illusion, memory flashback, illusion of familiarity, hallucination or illusion of self-image, and emotion; which are frequently evoked by temporal lobe stimulation or seizures.
- FT which originates in the frontal lobe may differ from FT of temporal lobe origin.
- The frontal lobe FT can be accompanied by an attempt to act on the thought (forced acts such as real behavior of the same content, vocalization, and gaze attraction), where it takes on colder and more ideational aspect, particularly more intentional, as thoughts that impose them and then need to find a way to materialize.
- FT of the temporal lobe origin requires the limbic system for expression. Therefore, the content of the FT is set in a much more intense and vivid experiential, emotional, and affective contexts

however the content of FT originating in the temporal lobe may be vaguer expression.

4. Ans. b. Amitriptyline

(Ref: A Short Textbook of Psychiatry, Ahuja, p200)

Amitriptyline, as in the question no other drug causes/responsible for TdP.

The widening of QRS and prolonged QT interval is both widely seen and associated with the potentially deadly rhythm, torsades de pointes (TdP).

Drugs causing torsades de pointes:

Antipsychotics	Antidepressants	Antihypertensive/ antiarrhythmics
❍ Chlorpromazine	❍ Amitriptyline	❍ Quinidine
❍ Haloperidol	❍ Doxepin	❍ Procainamide
❍ Droperidol	❍ Imipramine	❍ Disopyramide
❍ Quetiapine	❍ Nortriptyline	❍ Flecainide
❍ Olanzapine	❍ Desipramine	❍ Encainide
❍ Amisulpride	❍ Mianserin	❍ Sotalol
❍ Thioridazine	❍ Citalopram	❍ Amiodarone
❍ Pimozide—maximum risk	❍ Escitalopram	
	❍ Venlafaxine	
	❍ Bupropion	
	❍ Moclobemide	